mant:

Complaints:

ssity for Inpatient Care:

nt Illness:

RUNNING
WITH
GHOSTS

Medical History – General:

pitalizations/Surgery:

A MEMOIR OF SURVIVING
CHILDHOOD CANCER

dication

t:

ergies/Asthma:

uries (Fractures, etc.)

History (Pre-natal, Peri-natal, and Post-natal):   Birth Wt.:

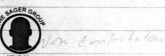

pmental History: Sitting: Standing: Walking:

king: Dentition   Toilet Training:

Running With Ghosts: A Memoir of Surviving Childhood Cancer
By Matt Tullis

Cover Design by: Stravinski Pierre and Siori Kitajima,
SF AppWorks LLC http://www.sfappworks.com
Formatting by Siori Kitajima and Ovidiu Vlad for SF AppWorks LLC
E-Book Formatted by Ovidiu Vlad

Cataloging-in-Publication data for this book
is available from the Library of Congress.

ISBN-13: 978-0-9980793-3-2
ISBN-10: 0-9980793-3-2

Published by The Sager Group LLC
info@TheSagerGroup.net
info@MikeSager.com

RUNNING WITH GHOSTS

A MEMOIR OF SURVIVING CHILDHOOD CANCER

BY MATT TULLIS

THE SAGER GROUP

Artifex Te Adiuva

For Alyssa, Emery, and Lily

But this too is true: Stories can save us.
—Tim O'Brien, *The Things They Carried*

Table of contents

Author's Note

This is not a memoir based solely on what I remember. When I first knew I wanted to write a book about this time in my life, one thing I realized early on was that my memory of those days in the hospital was not reliable.

As such, Part I of this book and parts of Part II have been built using my medical records, as well as interviews with many of the people I interacted with, including my parents, nurses, and, on one day in December 1997, Dr. Alex Koufos. Anything that appears in a quotation marks in Part I is an approximation of what most likely was said, based on the notes that my nurses recorded in their flow charts or based on a very clear rememberance on my part. Because some of the interviews I conducted were done more than a decade ago, I no longer have notes from many of these interviews, but I do still have many pieces that I wrote (but never published) based on those conversations. As for the medical records and the nursing flow charts, sometimes I was lucky and my nurses put my own words in quotation marks, although most often they didn't. They never put their own words in quotation marks, either, and so it is in those places, where I have created dialogue between a nurse and me, that I have approximated what was said.

Parts II and III are largely built on interviews or correspondence I have done with family members of my doctor, one of my nurses, and several patients I knew. Anything in quotation marks in these sections was either remembered by those being interviewed, was actually said by them to me, or showed up in the form of emails, letters, or other forms of correspondence.

I also utilized videos, newspaper articles, diaries, and and other writings done by the people I am writing about. Anywhere I mention what the weather was like, I have double-checked that in online archives. In short, I've tried to confirm that everything in this book is an accurate a portrayal of what happened to me and everyone I write about.

Prologue

hen I lace up my shoes to go for a run, I lace up the shoes of ghosts from a lifetime ago. When I strap on my watch, it transports me back to a different time, a time when my ghosts were alive, when we interacted and all faced the same unknown future. When I step out onto the road, they are there. Todd hobbles along, a prosthetic left leg replacing the one he lost when he was a little boy. Tim is there, and he is strong, able to keep up with no trouble thanks to the endless hours he spent in a pool as a high school swimmer. Melissa is there, especially when I run trails and have to be careful about picking my feet up high to avoid rocks and roots. We called it the stork walk in 1992, and it was necessary back then because our legs and feet were emaciated by the drugs designed to save us. Janet is there, with her runner's body, telling me about her children, who are close to my age, asking me how I am feeling and whether or not I am experiencing any pain. When I run with her, I am not. Finally, there is Dr. Alex Koufos. He is big and slow, but keeps churning on alongside me, whispering into my ear that my heart is strong, that I need to keep pushing forward, that the finish line is within reach.

I've run with my ghosts on back roads in rural Ohio, cutting through corn and soybean fields. I've run with them through the curving, hilly roads of southwest Connecticut, where I live now. I've run with them in the middle of the night in the middle of nowhere Kentucky, as rain was pounding down on me. I've run with them on the beaches of the Florida Gulf Coast and on the sidewalks of Traverse City, Michigan. I've run with them on the desert plains of north central Texas in late July. I've run with them in a foot of snow in February through a cemetery and an arboretum in Wooster, Ohio, and on those paths in the summer with my son and daughter as we raced a 5K together. I've run with them in the cold morning air of Indiana, just hours before my grandpa's funeral. I've run with them on the streets of Akron, during a marathon, where they pushed me forward, toward a finish line that sat in the shadow of Akron Children's Hospital, where we all came together a quarter-century ago, where I was saved and they were not.

I cling to my ghosts because they tie me to those days when my life was in the balance. It's a time I am continually drawn to as I try to understand more about my own life and how it was shaped by a random (or perhaps not) blip on my DNA, a chance mutation that threw everything into chaos. They were there in that chaotic time, suffering through their own chaotic lives, and I find myself thinking about them all the time. And yet, I often realize I know so little about them, as well as myself.

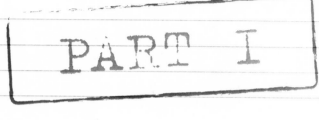

PART I

SICK COOKIE

CHAPTER 1

It Begins

I woke up on the morning of January 2, 1991, at 6 a.m. I always woke up at 6 a.m. I liked to get a quick shower and watch the news on channel 8. The weatherman—Andre Bernier, still a weatherman on that station—had a thing in the morning called Andre's Coffee Quiz. People throughout northeast Ohio sent in postcards with their names and phone numbers on them, and then each morning, Andre would draw a name out, call that person, and ask them a science-related question. If the person got the question right, they won fifty dollars and a coffee mug. When I was in the eighth grade, I sent a postcard in. A couple months later, he pulled my name. The question had something to do with what the basic element in plastic was. It was multiple-choice, but I didn't need the choices. I knew it was carbon. I got the fifty dollars and mug in the mail a couple days later.

I loved to watch Andre do the quiz, even though I was no longer eligible to participate. I had always enjoyed testing my knowledge against others, but I also liked watching the news, seeing what was going on in Cleveland and Akron, even though I lived about an hour south of the city on the lake and forty-five minutes southwest of Akron. There was something compelling to me, even as a young teen, about always knowing what was happening around me, and I was fascinated with the people who got to tell others that information.

I got dressed, pausing to consider what new Christmas clothes to wear on the first day back to school. I walked to the bus stop along with my brother John, who was in the eighth grade. As we walked, I started feeling tired again. I had been feeling tired a lot lately. My legs were sluggish and my eyes wanted to close. My head swam a bit, but I pushed on. The walk was about a half-mile from our house, and we were there in about fifteen minutes.

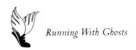

When we got to school, I hung out with my friends in the lobby. The space was huge, and all of the kids in the high school lounged about, standing on the marble floors or sitting on wooden benches that lined the walls on either side of both sets of doors. My friends and I had claimed a bench that we stood around early in our freshman year. It was right beside one of the doors that everyone walked through after getting off the bus or after parking cars. Rarely did anyone sit down on the bench. Instead, we stood—Jim (Pag to everyone), Doug, Ken, Bob, Jason, Josh, and me—and talked about what we did over break. I didn't mention the doctor's office visit on Friday, where our family doctor looked closely at the tiny red dots on my feet and ankles, pressed my back where I claimed it hurt, and ordered blood tests. Our primary objective on mornings like this was to just kill time with useless banter—making fun of each other, bragging about things we claimed to do but never did, that sort of thing—until the bell rang, when we would all walk off to our home rooms. This morning, that bell would signal the start of the second half of our freshman year.

While we were catching up, sweat started beading up on my forehead and my ears felt like they were on fire. I felt my head start swimming again. My vision went in and out. When it was in, it was blurry. I couldn't even see my friends, who were standing just a couple feet away from me. I felt like I was about to fall over. I stumbled around, looking for something solid to grab onto. My friends noticed and guided me down to a sitting position on the bench. I put my head between my knees, not because I knew I was passing out and that's what you do when you start to pass out, but because it seemed like the most logical thing to do. Slowly, my eyes started to focus again, and the dizziness left. While I no longer felt like I was about to end up on the floor, I was exhausted and wanted nothing more than to curl up on the bench and go to sleep.

The bell rang and my friends went to their classes, but not before I promised them I was all right. I waited for the lobby to clear and made my way, slowly, to the office, where I told the secretery I wasn't feeling good and needed to call my dad so he could come get me. Dad was at home but only for another couple of hours. He was a truck driver and had a load he was taking to South Bend, Indiana, later in the day. I walked back to the bench by the door and waited for Dad to pull up in his silver Mercury. When I saw him outside, I walked to the car. Every step was a chore. I was so tired, I just wanted to lie down on the sidewalk and fall asleep.

The fall of 1990 was hard for me. Sometime in September or October, Mom took me to a doctor to get a physical so I could play basketball on the freshman team. I wasn't very good, but I loved playing, and I loved being on the team. While baseball would always be my one, true, athletic love, basketball was certainly becoming my clear second-favorite sport. Unfortunately, when the doctor grabbed my scrotum and told me to turn my head and cough, he felt a bulge, a tiny spot where the lining had given way, and my intestines risked plunging down into my ball sack. I had a hernia, he said, and I wouldn't be playing basketball that year. Instead, I would be going under the knife of Dr. Walter Kerney.

And so I found myself entering Wooster Community Hospital just before Thanksgiving. Before surgery, though, my blood was drawn and tested. It was routine, just part of the surgical procedure. That blood work showed an elevated number of white blood cells in my body. It wasn't high enough to postpone the surgery, or even for a doctor to investigate further. Mom and I explained it away by the fact I had just had a cold. I had the surgery and was kept in the hospital for just about twenty-three hours, at which point I was discharged, not because I had recovered from the anesthesia—I was still vomiting up anything I ate—but because if they kept me any longer, I wouldn't be considered an outpatient, and that was not an option. I hobbled into the house, feeling every bit like a ninety-year-old man, hunched over and shuffling my feet, the two-inch incision in my lower-abdomen blazing with pain. But slowly, very slowly, I recovered from that surgery. A couple weeks later, my friends and I spent the night toilet-papering houses in the area, including the house of our vocational agriculture teacher. Right about the time I felt like I was back to normal, though, I started feeling like I wasn't. I had a cold I couldn't shake. My back started hurting. I was tired.

Had they looked more closely at those white blood cells before my surgery, they likely would have found immature cells, mutant cells that could not and would not fight infection in my body. Bone marrow makes all of the cells that come together to form our blood. It makes white cells, which fight infection; red cells, which carry oxygen to the body's organs; and platelets, which help clot the blood when it needs to be clotted. But sometimes, as in my case, something happens. This was the beginning. This was when my life changed, and it changed without anyone ever knowing. Somehow, my marrow started producing immature white cells—blasts—and stopped producing red cells and platelets. That's why my white count was elevated.

As we neared Christmas break at school, I found that the pain in my back was growing, and that I felt it in my side now. Every time I sneezed or coughed, it felt like I was being stabbed. If my brothers hit my back because we were fighting about something, I collapsed to the floor, spasms of pain shooting through my body. I came home from school each day and immediately fell asleep. We—my parents and I—rationalized it at home. I probably had mono, which explained why I was so tired. I probably broke a rib sneezing (which seems ridiculous, until you heard me sneeze) when I had that cold, the cold that wouldn't go away, and that explained the pain I felt.

We made the typical trips to southwest Ohio and Indiana to visit grandparents, aunts, and uncles over Christmas Break. One day, during the week between Christmas and New Year's, we went to a movie theater in Troy, Ohio, and watched *Home Alone* in a matinee showing. The theater was deserted because a massive snowstorm was blowing in. When we walked into the theater, there was no snow on the ground. When we walked out a couple hours later, there was at least five inches of snow on top of our car. As that snow belted down, we laughed at a young boy who had stymied two invaders who were trying to break into his house. Little did we know there were invaders inside my own body, mutant cells massing and planning an assault that would leave me alone and scared in a way I had never felt before. But we didn't know that, and for the movie's ninety minutes, I stopped feeling tired. I didn't concentrate on the pain in my back and side. I stopped feeling like there was something wrong with me. It would be the last normal thing I would do for a long time.

On the weekend after Christmas, we went to Indiana to visit my grandpa and Dottie. This was always one of my favorite trips because Dottie made the most amazing food—turkey, mashed potatoes, noodles, and more. The noodles were what I lived for every Christmas, that and all of her cookies: sugar cookies with icing and snicker doodles and chocolate chip and no-bake cookies. We could eat as much as we wanted. There was so much food, but there were also so many people. My dad has three brothers and two sisters, and by this trip, his youngest brother, Bob, and wife had already had their first daughter, and Kim was expecting another any day now. This was the one time a year when all of the Tullis cousins were gathered in one place, and because I was the oldest, I often set the tone, at least for the kids.

Except this year, I didn't eat anything. I didn't play with my cousins or brothers. I didn't even hang out in the living room and watch football with my uncles. Instead, I collapsed on the living room floor, smothered myself in the shag carpet and slept the entire day.

On New Year's Eve, a Monday, Mom took me to the doctor. This is the visit I didn't tell my friends about two days later at school, the visit where he asked funny questions and looked really closely at my feet and ankles, where he made sure I had more blood drawn. That night, I went to church, where the youth group was having a lock-in in the church gym. I had gone to these twice before, and they were so much fun I looked forward to them more than just about any other activity. We stayed up all night playing games, eating massive amounts of junk food, drinking Coke and Mountain Dew, and generally just being kids. But on this one, I curled up in a corner, covered myself with a coat, and went to sleep. I couldn't muster any energy at all, and I didn't know why. All I wanted to do was sleep and not move, lest pain shoot through my back.

I had been living for a month with my body fighting a war within itself. The mutant white cells had taken over. Very little oxygen was getting to my organs. Once the marrow became packed with the immature white cells, they were pushed out into the blood stream. Then they coagulated into a mass in my chest, which was the source of the pain in my back and side. The marrow just kept pumping out the mutants, over and over and over again. If I got sick, and I had been fighting a cold for what seemed like a month now, my body couldn't fight it off. I had bruises everywhere because my blood was flowing freely throughout my body. When the vessels broke in my legs and feet, something that happens all the time even in normal healthy people, the blood couldn't clot because there were no platelets, so I had tiny red pinprick dots all over the tops of my feet.

But I didn't know any of this. I knew my back hurt. I knew I was tired.

CHAPTER 2

First Night

It was just after 8 p.m., and I was sitting in a hospital bed and watching *Hoosiers*. The movie had come out in theatres about four years earlier. It was already a basketball classic, but I still hadn't seen it. Over the past couple of years I'd developed a love for the game, so I was excited when I learned the hospital had the movie in its VHS collection. As I watched, I was struck by how the buildings in the movie looked like ones I lived around, despite the fact I lived in small-town Ohio and the movie took place in small-town Indiana. Hickory High School looked a lot like Apple Creek Elementary School—the school I had gone to from kindergarten through the sixth grade—both in the exterior and interior shots. The barbershop where Gene Hackman's character meets all the men in the town looks like the place where Dad took me to get my hair cut. The movie felt like home, and at this point in time, I was aching for home.

Mom had gone back to our house to be with my younger brothers, John and Jim, for the night. Dad had gotten all the way to South Bend in his semi when he finally got the news that I was in the hospital. He was driving back now, as I sat and watched this movie and thought about what had happened during the course of the day, the strangest so far in my fifteen years.

Earlier in the day, I woke up from a long nap at around 1:30 p.m. Dad had left for South Bend shortly after he brought me home from school. Mom came home from work and took me to Dr. Frank Cebul's office in Wooster. I was feeling better, a bit rested, but that feeling always waned quickly, or at least lately it had been. But when we got to the doctor's office, we didn't go to an exam room. Instead, we went to the doctor's actual office and sat in chairs facing him as he sat behind a desk. Dr. Cebul said the results from my blood work, taken two days earlier, had come back, which was why he wanted to see us. Eventually, he asked me to step out into the hallway, and he talked to Mom alone. I don't know how long they were in there. Five minutes. Ten. Fifteen. Eventually, Mom came out and said we needed to go to the hospital for some more tests. She promised me pizza later that evening. In the minivan, as we made the short drive to the hospital, she said something about leukemia, but I didn't know what that was and didn't ask. I thought maybe she had actually said Lou Gerhig's, as in the disease that struck down one of the greatest baseball players of all time. I loved baseball. I thought it would be cool to have the same problem as Gehrig, which just goes to show I didn't know anything about his disease or leukemia or anything other than the fact that I wanted to play basketball that weekend and I wanted pizza for dinner.

I imagined I would be in the hospital for a short amount of time. Maybe a day. I would have some tests done and then go home. But I was immediately admitted, at 2:20 p.m., to room 404 in the pediatric wing of the hospital. A nurse walked into the room shortly after I got settled in the bed and started talking to Mom. The nurse had long brown hair, glasses. She looked like she was about Mom's age. She was quiet and acted like she was used to dealing with much younger patients than someone like me, a teenager.

Eventually, she started asking Mom questions from a piece of paper. At one point, Mom said I had been exposed to mono sometime in the previous four weeks. She also mentioned my hernia surgery in November and told the nurse that I was nauseated after the surgery.

"How do you feel as a parent?" the nurse asked.

"Okay," Mom said.

"Why did you bring your child to the hospital?" she asked.

"He's tired," Mom said. "He's not eating as much. He says his back and side hurts."

I had also lost three pounds in the last week, Mom said.

"What have you told your child about coming to the hospital?" the nurse asked.

"Nothing," Mom said, although that wasn't entirely truthful. "The doctor just said he needed to be admitted."

Mom left the hospital around 3:30, but returned at 5 and brought Little Caesars pizza with her. I ate several pieces and drank a Coke, the second one of the day. I didn't often get to drink Coke, and here it was being freely offered, so I took it. I talked on the phone with my friend Pag and told him I was in the hospital, but that I expected I would still play in the Future Farmers Association club basketball tournament over the weekend. I had been looking forward to that tournament ever since I found out I couldn't play on the freshman team because of the hernia surgery.

It was the talk of basketball with Jim and my hopes that I would play that weekend that pulled me into *Hoosiers*. I tried to concentrate on the movie, but now that I was alone, I started getting nervous. I had spent a night in this hospital before—just about a month and a half ago—when I had my hernia surgery, but this just seemed different. Then, I entered the hospital early in the morning, had surgery, and spent time in a room I shared with a high school classmate who had surgery on his broken nose. I spent most of that day throwing up. Nurses kept giving me toast and telling me I couldn't go home until I kept food down.

But now I was in a room by myself, and nobody was talking about going home. Dr. Cebul had also sent in a new doctor who I had never seen before, Dr. Jeffrey Spiess, an oncologist, although I didn't know what that meant, and this man talked more about leukemia. He talked about all the tests I would have the following day—more blood tests and something about bone marrow.

"Then we'll know more," he probably said. "We'll know where we go from here."

Additionally, Pastor Don, the youth pastor at my church, stopped by the hospital just after I finished eating. I loved Pastor Don. He was so different from any of the other preachers I had ever met. He was young and related to the teens in our church at a time when I had just become one. He asked me how I was feeling, and truthfully, I felt fine at that moment. I felt rested. My stomach was full. That's what was so confusing. I didn't feel like someone who should be stuck in a hospital bed, at least not at that exact moment. But I also knew, deep down, that something was wrong.

As I watched the boys from a small town in Indiana play basketball for a school that wasn't much bigger than the one I went to, I wondered what was happening to me. My nerves kicked in, and I started twirling the long curly hair at the back of my head with my left hand. The room was dark, just a fluorescent light affixed to the wall above my bed. I liked to watch movies with the lights off, and so the only light was the buzzing fluorescent and the glow off the television as Gene Hackman tried to teach these boys who looked like men how to play basketball, how to be a team, how to slay giants. I liked the darkness for the movie, but it also amplified the loneliness. I could see bright white lights outside my hospital room. The entire place was quiet—the only sound coming from the musical montages of the boys from Hickory winning basketball games—a complete departure from my previous stay, when saws and drills and jackhammers, sounds of construction, flooded the room I constantly vomited in.

Around 8 p.m., the nurse came into my room and sat down in a chair beside my bed. It had been at least five hours since she had asked Mom those questions. I glanced at her but then looked back at the television. She asked me how I was feeling, and I mumbled that I was fine. I cracked my knuckles, all of them multiple times.

"Why do you do that?" she asked.

"They hurt if I don't," I said.

Earlier, before Mom left, the nurse told us that if we had any questions about any of the upcoming tests, we just had to ask. Now that Mom was gone, I didn't have any questions. Or rather, I had hundreds of questions, but none of them had answers, or at least none that I figured could be answered now. Why was I here? When was I going home? What is leukemia? What is bone marrow? Will I ever play basketball or baseball again? Does this have anything to do with my surgery from a month ago? What is wrong with me?

I focused on the movie to push those thoughts out of my head. I thought that if I could pay attention to the boys from Hickory and see if they could really win a state championship against a big city school, then I would be fine. Everything would be fine. But my mind kept wandering to the creeping loneliness of this hospital room and the feeling that my life was changing in ways I could never imagine.

Tears rolled down my face as I looked at the TV. I didn't say anything and neither did the nurse. She sat there quietly. Had she left, I would have begged her to come back into the room, but she didn't, and the loneliness and fears lifted, if only for a short time.

I stayed awake until after midnight. I didn't want to close my eyes because I didn't know what would when I opened them. Every so often, I started crying again, worried about what was going on, but then I pulled myself together, or at least tried to. I dried my face. I stared at the television, which now was playing who knows what, and figured if I could just focus, everything would be all right. And it was, until it wasn't, and the tears flowed again.

The nurse came back into my room around midnight and sat with me for a moment. She asked how I was feeling and said that if I had any questions, I simply had to ask them. I insisted I didn't have any questions, that I was fine. But the tears in my eyes betrayed me, and she made note of them in her nursing notes. Eventually, I fell asleep.

There was a dull push into my left hip. Then harder. Harder. There was a grinding as Dr. Spiess pushed a six-inch-long, thick needle into the bone. But I didn't really feel anything, just the pushing and the grinding as the needle pierced me and sank into the marrow of my hip bone. While Dr. Spiess started pulling out the soft, spongy, fatty tissue that hung out inside my bones, I was floating above the bed, asleep but not really asleep, aware but not really aware. Before he had wiped down a spot on my skin with an alcohol swab and injected Novocain, a nurse had pushed Demerol into the IV port on the top of my left hand. So he pushed and grinded and sucked the marrow out of me, and I was just there, the drug rendering me into near bliss.

I woke up at about 9:30 a.m., about thirty minutes after Dr. Spiess had done the bone marrow aspiration. Mom was no longer at my bedside, as she had been when the procedure started. She was, at that moment, driving to Akron Children's Hospital with the marrow sample, which Dr. Spiess had given to her to deliver, where it would be tested.

"You will get it there much faster than a courier service," he told her.

Speed, he said, was of the essence.

I lay on my back in my hospital bed, a bunch of gauze and tape on my hip.

"You have to stay on your back for about forty minutes," a nurse, a different nurse than the one who had sat with me the night before, said to me.

I didn't move. I had no idea what was going on. I craved the feeling the drugs had given me earlier, but I didn't ask for more. I wondered where Mom was. Or Dad. Had I seen him since he dropped me off at the house the day before? Grandma McEowen walked into my room around 11 a.m., and I was happy to see someone I knew, but also confused as to why she was in Wooster. She lived more than three hours away. This was all so weird and confusing.

The day before, after a nurse pulled blood out of my arm, someone in a room at Wooster Community Hospital put a drop on a slide and smeared it, then slid that slide into a hemocytometer, which counted the white blood cells, red blood cells, platelets, and more in the sample. There were 139,000 white blood cells. The normal amount of white blood cells is 10,000.

Now, in Akron, someone was looking at a small clot, less than 0.1 cc, of my bone marrow and seeing that all of the spaces in the tissue were filled to capacity with leukemic cells. Dr. Spiess saw the results and called the nurses' station on my floor in Wooster. He ordered a chest x-ray.

"And we need a copy of his chart to be made for transfer to Akron Children's Hospital," he said.

A short while later, Dr. Spiess told Mom that I was going to be moved to Akron, possibly that evening. He said the hospital there had a hematology and oncology clinic that was far more adept at handling the disease that I had—and I did have leukemia, acute lymphoblastic leukemia to be exact—than a small hospital in Wooster could.

Later that evening, around 6 p.m., Dr. Spiess told Mom that I would instead be transferred in the morning, but that she and Dad could drive me. He told Mom that I was incredibly sick. I had a mass in my chest where mutant white cells had gathered. That is what had caused the pains I felt in my back and side. He said I had no immune system, no platelets to clot my blood should I be cut.

Later, Mom relayed to me some of what Dr. Spiess had said. It all seemed so foreign, so out of the blue. "I'm scared," I told her.

I knew that she was too.

CHAPTER 3

The First Meeting

kron Children's Hospital. 4-North. Room 462. That's where I found myself two days after watching *Hoosiers*. There were two beds in the room, but I was, and would be, the only patient there for the next ten weeks. I chose the bed beside the window, which looked out at the intersection of West State and Locust streets. It's a four-way stop now, but at the time, there was a blinking traffic light, with a yellow light for the vehicles traveling on West State Street and a red blinking light for those on Locust. Across State Street was the Ronald McDonald House. Four floors below me was the emergency room, and so my parents often watched ambulances pull in with sirens blaring and lights flashing. Outside my door, there was the nurses' station, a big, long desk that ran the length of about five or six hospital rooms. Running along either side of that desk were two long hallways that, in the coming weeks, Dad would occasionally force me to walk to get a little bit of exercise.

There was a bathroom with a shower near the doorway to my room. Across from my bed, a television was mounted on the wall. Below the television, a large bulletin board that would come to be cluttered with the more than 150 get-well cards I would receive. There was a windowsill that would also become cluttered, with boxes of baseball cards and flowers in a Pittsburgh Steelers vase and more. But now it was empty. Everything in the room was bare. It was just me, my parents, and a hospital room with a television and a window onto the world, a window that I would eventually view as a barrier, as something I could, or rather would, never get beyond.

We got to Akron Children's around 9:30 a.m. on January 4, a Friday. After about an hour, an orderly showed up with a wheelchair. I had never needed a wheelchair before, but I sat in it, and for the first time since I was a baby, before I could walk, I relied on someone else to move me from point A (the third-floor lobby) to point B (the fourth floor). By 10:40, I was getting settled in the bed by the window and a nurse was showing Mom and Dad everything in the room—the closet, the bathroom, the call buttons. At 1:30 p.m., another bone marrow biopsy was done, but already, the blissful high of the Demerol was diminished. I didn't feel as though I was floating as high. I didn't feel pain, but the pleasure of the drug was less than it had been just one day earlier. By 3 p.m. I was asleep, and Mom and Dad were sitting beside the bed, watching the television, watching me, talking to family members and friends on the phone. It was a scene that would come to be the most common one in the next three months: Matt "quietly resting" or "asleep" with "parents at bedside," a scene nurses would note hundreds of times. But this was the first, at least in Akron.

I met Dr. Alex Koufos for the first time that evening when he visited with Mom, Dad, and me at 7 p.m. He introduced himself and talked a bit about what we—what I—was facing. He looked directly at me most of the time, although he also made eye contact with my parents. He asked a lot of questions: How I was feeling, When did I start feeling sick? He asked me to describe how I felt. What parts of my body hurt? How often was I tired? I wasn't overly responsive. I was dazed, unsure of what was happening. I was awake for this visit, but also off in another world. Because I couldn't answer the questions, Mom stepped in. She told Dr. Koufos that about four weeks ago, I had a cold. I was coughing a lot, had nasal congestion and a sore throat. And that cold persisted. Then about two weeks ago, it morphed. I stopped eating and complained that I felt like I was going to throw up. I was constantly tired.

Eventually, Dr. Koufos put his stethoscope to my chest, but not before apologizing for its coldness, and listened to my heart and my lungs. He felt my abdomen, pressing his large hands deep against my skin. That's when he felt the enlarged spleen and liver. He checked my eyes, ears, and throat.

When he was done, he told us that the results from the most recent bone marrow biopsy would be in the next day. The results, he said, would give us a clearer understanding of exactly what type of cancer, what type of leukemia, I was battling, and that, he said, would help him know how to fight it.

Earlier that day, just after eight ccs of bone marrow was pulled out of my left hip bone, a nurse started me on an IV of sodium bicarbonate, which is basically baking soda. Sodium bicarbonate would increase my body's pH level. The purpose was to prepare me for the upcoming barrage of toxic drugs that would be pumped into my body. This truly was the first move, the first offensive maneuver, in the battle that was about to explode inside of me. It was the declaration of war, a signal to the invading, mutant white blood cells that bombs were coming, and they were going to be devastating.

Early the next day, a Saturday morning, Dr. Koufos got the results from the bone marrow biopsy, and he sat down to write in his Physician's Progress Record.

"Matt is a 15-year-old white male who presents with three-week history of fatigue, back and leg pain," he wrote. "He was noted to have a peripheral blood count of 110,000. Chest X-ray revealed a mediastinal mass. Referred for further evaluation. Physical exam reveals a spleen of three centimeters, liver enlarged to four centimeters. LAB reveals a total WBC of 149,000 white 86 percent BLAST."

In just one day, I had gone from 110,000 to 149,000 white blood cells in the sample of blood taken from me. And 86 percent of those cells were immature. They were the leukemic cells. And my bone marrow? Nearly all of the cells in the marrow were leukemic. It was packed full of mutant cells, cells that, if left untreated, would kill me in just a couple weeks.

Later that day, we sat in a conference room off the nurses' station on 4-North. Dr. Koufos was on one side of the table. Mom and Dad were on the other side, and I sat at the end, so the three most important adults in my life at that moment flanked me. There were binders sitting on the table, big white binders that were full of papers. But we were focused on a five-page document titled "Children's Hospital Medical Center of Akron in affiliation with Children's Cancer Study Group Informed Consent."

The meeting lasted for more than an hour, and I said very little. I was silent. Mom listened to everything Dr. Koufos said while simultaneously freaking out over my lack of engagement. She looked at me and saw someone who had checked out, who had already given up. It was like I wasn't even there.

And perhaps I wasn't, mentally at least. We were in a well-lit room just off the nurse's station, and yet I felt like it was dark, like a spotlight was shining on the table, on those binders. I was there, but I wasn't, floating above everyone else in the room as they discussed exactly what was happening inside my body—the mutant leukemic white blood cells taking over everything, forming the mass in my chest, causing some of my organs to become enlarged, making it so there were no red cells to carry oxygen, no platelets to stop internal bleeding, and no functional white cells to fight infections—and what was going to happen to my body, not just over the next day or two, but over the next 785 days. More than two years. He told us about the way I was going to be assaulted by chemicals and drugs I had never heard of. I was going to be irradiated. I was going to be destroyed, leveled, because the only way to defeat a cancer of the blood is to kill everything, all of the cells, the good ones and the bad ones, and hope that the marrow is shocked into making the right cells again.

We were in a haze, listening to Dr. Koufos speak for a long time in his soft, careful, measured tones. Mom and Dad nodded. Mom asked questions and Dad sat there, stunned, refusing to think that anything could ever be this bad. That this was a joke. That everything would be all right because he had a remarkable feeling about this doctor, this man who was laying out what was undoubtedly a horrific and frightening plan to save my life, but that it would work.

The document we spent the most time on described a treatment study I would be enrolled in, if we agreed. While everything Dr. Koufos had said regarding what had happened to me so far, and what lie ahead, surely frightened Mom and Dad to some extent, the third paragraph of this consent form was the most sobering thing my parents had heard since I entered the hospital three days earlier in Wooster.

"You/your child has acute lymphoblastic leukemia which has been characterized as having a poor prognosis or outlook on standard therapy. This means that within the group, some children have the potential for cure and others may not respond well to treatment or the duration of remission (control of disease) may be relatively short."

For the first time, my parents realized I might die.

The second page of the document details the treatment plan and how the two protocols, which I would be randomly placed in one of them, differed.

"This protocol incorporates the best currently known therapy for this form of leukemia," Dr. Koufos read to us. "Half of the children will receive additional intensive therapy which is of an investigative nature in an attempt to improve on previous results."

We could not know which treatment I would get, and after Dr. Koufos got to page 3 and started discussing side effects, my parents were potentially frightened by the possibility of my getting "additional intensive therapy," or any treatment. But what option was there?

"What if we don't want to do the study," Mom asked Dr. Koufos.

If Mom and Dad didn't sign off on the study, Dr. Koufos said, then I would receive what was currently the standard treatment, which still included just about all of the drugs we were looking at. The difference, he said, was the timing and duration. No matter what we chose, Dr. Koufos said, I would be given drugs that would make me incredibly sick. But it was the only way to save my life.

Mom and Dad looked at the document where the drugs and their side effects were listed.

"Cyclophosphamide: Low blood counts, nausea and vomiting, hair loss, blood in urine, lowered sperm count."

"Vincristine: Irritation of the tissues if the drug leaks into the tissue during intravenous administration, jaw and abdominal pain, hair loss, constipation, decreased reflexes and poor neuromuscular coordination, muscle weakness, numbness or tingling, urine retention, bone marrow depression and convulsions."

"Methotrexate: Low blood counts, mouth sores, diarrhea, rash. Temporary mild abnormalities of liver, kidney, lung function may be noted. Headache, stiff neck, convulsions, decrease in intellectual function when given in the spinal fluid."

They went on, and on, and on.

But without these treatments, I would die. And soon. My body could have held out for another couple weeks. If we did nothing, I would get more and more tired. I would stop moving and perhaps slip into a coma. The mutant white cells would invade every crevice inside my body, and eventually they would shut down all of my organs. I would die in my sleep, my body overrun by an invader.

That, clearly, was not an option.

Dr. Koufos gave us the paper, and we went back to my hospital room. A nurse hooked me back up to my IV, and then Mom and Dad considered the possibilities, which had essentially come down to whether or not to enroll me in the study. No matter what they chose, I was still going to get dangerous drugs pumped into my body. They chose the study. I was no longer thinking clearly or even deeply about what was happening. During that meeting, I separated my brain from my body. I pulled away and viewed myself as another, as someone I was watching all of this happen to.

Mom and Dad signed the informed consent form on Monday morning, two days after the meeting, and just before I headed in for surgery to install a central line in my chest. The central line was a decision we made in that meeting with Dr. Koufos, and the one thing I actually remember participating in. The choices were to have a line come out of my chest that nurses could hook IVs up to as well as draw blood from, versus a port just under the skin. The upside to the latter was it could get wet, and thus I could still go swimming and take showers. The thought of needles pulled me out of my haze. It was a pain I was aware of, had experienced, and I wanted to avoid it. I shuttered at the thought of my skin being pierced constantly, so I chose the central line. I didn't realize it would require dressing changes every four days, which would make me fear water for the next two years.

Just before the surgery, which was performed by Dr. David Andrews, at 9 a.m., Pastor Don from the church youth group spent time by my bed. He had visited a couple of times already, always praying with me, or more accurately for me, before he left. Now, as a nurse pushed anesthesia into the IV that currently ran through my hand but would soon run through my chest, he asked me if I wanted to pray, to ask God to come into my heart. The anesthesia was already starting to make my brain swirl, but I shook my head yes at Pastor Don because I liked him so much and, even then as a fifteen-year-old, I was still fearful of dying without God in my heart because I didn't want to go to hell. As Pastor Don prayed for my life, both my physical life and my spiritual one, as he asked God to take me safely through the surgery and to deliver me from this disease that was eating up the insides of my body, as he asked God and Jesus to take up residence in my heart, my world went black.

CHAPTER 4

The Purge

I woke up and opened my eyes. My throat hurt. My chest ached. My bladder felt like it was about to explode. What day was it? What time? I looked out the window, but it was gray, lots of clouds filling the small slice of sky that I could see.

"I have to pee."

The words creaked out of my mouth, barely able to escape my cracked lips.

Mom stood up from the chair she was sitting in, which was between my bed and the window. She walked to the end of the bed and grabbed the plastic jug that hung on a bedrail. Then she lowered the rail on the left side of my bed and helped me stand up. She held the plastic tubes that were dangling from the IV pole and snaking their way up my T-shirt and into my chest. They felt like chains, tethering me to the bed. I put weight on my legs, but they were weak, a Jell-O incapable of holding anything upright. It seemed like it took hours for me to actually get on my feet, but it was only just seconds, thirty maybe, but a brief realization flashed through my mind, one that told me I could no longer do something that less than a week ago had been so simple. After another few seconds, I was steady on my feet, and Mom handed me the jug. She pulled a curtain around my bed so I could have some privacy. I uncapped the jug, pulled down the shorts I was wearing—they were cut-offs, were once big, baggy green, MC Hammer style pants that I wore in the eighth grade—and pushed my penis into the open mouth of the jug and starting pissing. It was one of the greatest feelings of my life.

The urine poured out of me in a frothy stream. It was dark orange and stunk far worse than anything I had ever pissed or shit out of my body before. I stood there and felt the bottle get warmer and warmer as the urine came closer to the top. When I was done, I had emptied nearly thirty ounces of seemingly toxic urine into the bottle.

"I'm done," I said to Mom, my bladder feeling better, but my body still feeling like it was on fire.

She opened the curtain, took the jug, and hung it on the end of the bed. There, it would wait for a nurse, who would log its volume, record its color, and test its acidity. Mom helped me lie back down in bed, which was far easier than getting out.

"Do you want anything?" she asked.

I asked her what day it was. It was Tuesday, she said. January 8. I had been in the hospital for almost a week now. Two days in Wooster and now four in Akron. The central line had been installed in my chest the day before, and the chemotherapy drugs had started being pumped into my body not long after I got out of surgery. Since then, I had woken up only a handful of times, always when I needed to piss. I often expelled, or voided, as the nurses liked to note, about seventy ounces of urine every eight hours. The urine, that gross, orange toxic filth that poured out of me, was a byproduct of the war that was raging inside my body. The drugs killed the cancer cells, and just about everything else it came into contact with, and what wasn't absorbed back into my body found its way filtered through my liver and kidneys and into my bladder. I was pissing the cancer out of me.

"What time is it?" I asked Mom.

I needed to know so I could change the channel on the television.

It was just after 4 p.m., she said.

I grabbed the remote and switched it to channel 43 so I could watch *DuckTales*. Then I settled back into the bed, fought back the rising nausea in my stomach, and closed my eyes.

How often did this happen? In my memory it seems like it happened hundreds of times, but it probably didn't happen more than five. Maybe ten. In my memory I feel like I was always sleeping, but my medical records from those first few days show that I wasn't always asleep. But that is what has stuck with me, the memories of the time when I wasn't in pain, when I could drift off and just for a few moments feel like everything was like it was a week ago, a month ago. Because when I woke up, it was all too real. There were IVs beeping when the chemo or the fluids ran dry. There were sirens outside. There were people coming into and out of my room every hour. There were Mom and Dad on the phone, updating everyone on my situation. I sought solace in the things that made me feel normal: sleep and my regular television-viewing pattern. And even then, that often wasn't enough.

The next morning, Janet Creech-Forrer walked into room 462. It was 8 a.m., the start of her shift. She introduced herself and made small talk. She asked where we were from, and when Mom told her we lived in Apple Creek, she said that she lived in Orrville. We had actually moved from southwest Ohio when I was four years old to Apple Creek because Dad's job as a truck driver was moved to Orrville. After a few years apart from that company, he had recently gone back to work there. All of the loads that he took to cities east and west of Ohio originated in the same small city my new nurse lived in. All of this information was exchanged with Janet, plus the fact that when I was little, we used to go to the Orrville Public Library. I had a birthday party at the McDonald's in Orrville once. It's the type of small talk that people who are meeting each other for the first time make once they realize they have a connection. In this case, it was even more important because now we, or at least Mom and Dad, knew that I had a nurse who understood where we were coming from and how frightening it was to be in a big city compared with the small towns we inhabited.

Janet did her normal check-up on me, the first of hundreds she would do over the next ten weeks. She took my blood pressure and recorded it as 108 over 48. She checked my pulse, and wrote down that my heart was beating eighty times every minute. She put a thermometer in my mouth, which eventually told her that my body temperature was 98.2 degrees.

I was lying in bed through all of this. Mom was in the chair beside my bed, which is where she almost always was, and Dad was sitting on the edge of the empty bed to my left. I told Janet I felt like I was going to throw up. She asked me what day it was and what time it was, although by this point, there was still no clock in the room. Still, I could tell what time it was by what was on television, and she noted that I was "alert and oriented to person, date and time." She checked the insides of my mouth and noted that it was pale pink and moist. She checked my central line and noticed a little bit of bright red blood oozing from where the line went into my chest. She checked my lungs and noted that I was breathing easily and that my lungs sounded clear.

Janet visited my room seventeen more times that day. She came in every time a doctor visited, first at 8:20 a.m. when Dr. Koufos came to look at the oozing blood near my central line. She came in again at 9:40 a.m. when

Dr. Andrews, the man who installed the central line just two days earlier, looked at the oozing that was soaking through the bandage.

Andrews said the dressing needed to be changed, so Janet came into my room with alcohol wipes, iodine and cotton swabs, as well as gauze and medical tape. She helped me pull my sweat-stained T-shirt off my already shrinking upper body. I lay back and she started to work, gently pulling at the tape that held the dressing in place, using alcohol wipes to losen the adhesive. It was tedious, something Mom and Dad would both have to learn how to do, but Janet made quick work of it. Once the tape was off, she gently lifted off the gauze dressing itself. Now, the bright red blood was much more noticeable, so she cleaned it up.

The central line went into the right side of my chest, just above my pectoral muscles, in a hole that would remain relatively open until the line was pulled out. That's why the dressing was necessary. She swabbed iodine around that entry point and then wiped it all down with alcohol before placing a new piece of gauze, which had a hole cut into it so the line could slide through, over the entry point. Then she taped me up nice and tight, and I slid my nasty T-shirt back on.

Janet and Dr. Koufos wanted to get me up and moving. The more time I spent in bed, the more muscle mass I would lose. The more muscle mass I lost, the harder my body would take the chemotherapy treatments. Janet asked if I wanted to get up and take a bath, but I said no. She asked if she could wash my hair at least, which was also becoming nasty. I said she could, as long as I didn't have to get out of bed. So she got some shampoo and had a little bit of water in a container by my bed, and she slowly started working the shampoo through what was still my long, brown hair.

When I first found out, in that meeting with Dr. Koufos, that my hair would fall out, I found that more frightening than anything else. I had long, thick, curly hair that fell almost to my shoulders, at least on the back of my head. I loved how it flowed out of the back of my baseball cap, how when I ran it blew behind me. I liked how my hair was there when I was nervous. I would reach back with my left hand and twirl my hair, tangling it up and then untangling it. I didn't want to lose my hair, and two days in, it was still holding strong.

I felt a little better after my hair had been washed. Even though I had only known Janet for just about two-and-a-half hours, I liked her and I wanted to impress her. So when she asked me to at least get out of bed, to sit in the chair that Mom usually sat in, for a few minutes, I agreed to do so.

Again, like the day before, when I stood to piss, and like every time I stood to piss, standing up was getting more difficult every time I did it. But Mom and Janet helped me stand up, and then I took a step or two over to the chair and sat down. While I sat and watched TV, an orderly came in and changed the sheets and blankets on my bed. Less than fifteen minutes later, though, I was back in bed.

Janet asked me how I was feeling after I climbed back into bed.

"I'm feeling bad," I said.

I hadn't eaten anything all day, had only drank a few ounces of water, and yet I was constantly pissing. In three hours, I filled a one-liter jug with orange urine.

But that wasn't all that was coming out of me.

Dr. Koufos came in to visit with Mom, Dad, and me around 11:30 a.m. Throughout his visit, I moaned and moved about my bed as though some invisible creature were torturing me. That's when I felt the bubbling in my stomach, a gurgling, the first feelings of a stomach that is about to turn itself inside out. I had already thrown up once that morning, a vomit that consisted of green stomach bile and little else. I didn't know how I could possibly puke again. I wretched. Nothing. I felt the acid climbing up the pipes from my stomach to my mouth, and I wretched again. Nothing. Then that acidic taste touched the back of my tongue, and I grabbed the tan, kidney-shaped bowl that sat on my bedside table. I wretched with every muscle left in my abdomen, and a little bit of green, followed by red, some blood, dribbled out of my mouth. I did it again, and a few more drops splashed into the bowl.

Throughout the day, Janet gave me nine different medications. I received a heavy dose of cyclophosphamide, a drug related to mustard gas that causes low blood counts, nausea, vomiting, hair loss, and blood in the urine, among other things. She also gave me prednisone, a steroid that I had to take in pill form. That drug was far more bitter to me than the cyclophosphamide, which I couldn't taste as it infused into my body through the central line. The prednisone pills left a horrible taste on my tongue if I couldn't swallow them quickly enough, and I never could because they were so big and my throat was so sore. I also received medication for my nausea, medication that didn't ultimately do much. I received Benadryl, although I don't know why. I received medication to prepare my body to receive a platelet infusion. And I received platelets.

Throughout the rest of the day, I ate nothing. I drank nothing. And yet I pissed another liter of urine that was filled with dead cancer cells. I was as miserable as I had ever been in my life, and I would have been more miserable had I known that it would get worse. Janet kept coming because it was her job, but also because she wanted to make sure I was all right.

At 3 p.m. I was awake, but I felt that twisting and bubbling in my stomach.

"I think I'm going to puke," I told Janet.

Twenty minutes later, and just forty minutes before Janet's shift was up and she could head back home to her husband and children in Orrville, ending her first day of taking care of me, I stood up to piss and started dripping blood. It was bright red and came from my central line. Janet came into the room and cleaned me up. Then, as she was clocking out and heading home, another nurse changed the dressing yet again and found a small blood clot at the spot where the central line went into my chest. She cleaned the clot out and put some medication around the line and bandaged me back up. I was fine after that. My evening was uneventful. I didn't vomit the rest of the night. I didn't bleed from anywhere. I continued to receive a lot of drugs. I watched television. I slept.

As I got to know many of the different nurses, I developed preferences. There were nurses I looked forward to seeing in my room, even if I was feeling horrible, and there were nurses I wanted nothing to do with (mostly just a third-shift nurse who always smelled like cigarette smoke). One of those nurses who made the days just a little more bearable was Theresa. She had the biggest and loudest laugh I had ever heard. She had a habit of doing anything it took to make a kid laugh.

She started calling me Bugle Boy, because one day she walked into my room and I was eating those Bugle corn snack chips. I was taking them out of the bag and placing them on the ends of my fingers, then pulling them off my fingers and into my mouth one by one. I also wore exactly two T-shirts while I was in the hospital, both with the Bugle Boy jeans logo on them. Once she gave me the nickname, I could tell when she was heading to my room from the nurses' station because I would hear her voice, all the way out in the hallway, sing, "Oh, Bugle Boyyyyyyyyyy!"

Theresa worked first shift with Janet, which meant that I usually had one of my two favorite nurses taking care of me when I woke up in the morning. Janet made me feel that I was her number one priority, and that no matter how bad things were, she was there to make them bearable and to give comfort when making something bearable didn't seem possible. While my own mom was there constantly (and if Mom wasn't, Dad was), Janet felt like a mom as well, and even better, she felt like a mom who could understand what I was experiencing. She didn't seek to make me laugh like Theresa did, but that wasn't necessarily her way. She nurtured. She sat and talked. In so many ways, she reminded me of the nameless nurse from Wooster, who sat with me as I cried through *Hoosiers*, a night that seemed so far in the past like it was a completely different life.

Janet would sometimes come into my room in the mornings, even if she wasn't my nurse for the day, just to say hi. Other times, when she was my nurse, there would be moments when she had to stay in my room for fifteen or thirty minutes, particularly after I had been given a certain drug, so she could watch for allergic reactions or bad side effects. When we had that extended time with her, we would talk about Orrville, which was about fifteen minutes from our house in Apple Creek. A lot of Saturdays in my childhood were spent at the factory where my Dad kept his truck. While Dad worked on his truck, or washed it, or whatever it was he did, my brothers and I rode Big Wheels and then later bicycles around the vast parking lot. Mom sat on a blanket on the ground and watched us. Sometimes, we had a picnic of turkey or ham sandwiches. If we had the money, we went to a restaurant in the city's downtown called Good Times, which had pizza, and, even better, popcorn that they brought to your table while you waited for your pizza. As I lie in a hospital bed thirty-five miles away from my real bed, Mom and Dad drove through Orrville every time they made the trip from Apple Creek to Akron. We had a lot of connections to the town, and because Janet lived there, we made a connection with her, and I think she connected with us. That's why, I imagine, she often stopped by my room just to see how I was doing.

I wasn't doing well, especially in those first two weeks of chemotherapy. The treatments for leukemia in 1991 had evolved dramatically from just two decades before, when doctors shot massive doses of radiation at a body and then gave one drug to the patients. In the late 1970s and '80s, doctors started experimenting by treating kids with leukemia with several different types of drugs all at once, something called combination chemotherapy. They knew the drugs would, when working together, kill the cancer cells. What they needed to figure out, though, was just how much patients could take. They needed to know how much they could give a patient and not kill them with the treatment because chemotherapy is some seriously bad shit.

Today, researchers and doctors are developing targeted drugs that kill only cancer cells, but in 1991, the treatments killed virtually all the cells they came into contact with. They didn't distinguish between good red blood cells and bad, mutant white blood cells. In many ways, it was like a carpet-bombing of an enemy's territory. Civilians were going to be killed, and you just had to live with those consequences.

One of the first casualties in this war was my appetite. I didn't want to eat, ever. The day after I started chemotherapy, I refused to eat lunch and then dinner. The smells of the food made me nauseous. I couldn't stand the thought of taking the lid off the tray. Even if I had eaten the food, I likely would have puked it up. I often vomited six or seven times a day. It would start with a rumbling in my stomach, even if there was no food there. Nausea would wash over me, and the next thing I knew I was retching. My vomit was like everything else that came out of my body—my piss and my shit—recorded by my nurses both in amount and color. Of course, everything that went in was also recorded in depth: the medicine, the food (or lack of food), the drink, which early on mostly consisted of water. Everything was carefully tracked. I ate a bag of Doritos once, and then thirty minutes later, I vomited, and it was orange with flecks of red.

My weight plummeted in those first few weeks. The day I started treatment, I weighed 127.9 pounds. Less than three weeks later, I weighed 101.9. It was the job of the first-shift nurse to weigh me every morning, and so Janet had that duty more than most. The worst part about it was the fact that it meant standing up. When Janet, or any other nurse, entered my room for the first time on first shift, they did so wheeling a scale. Janet would ask how I was feeling and then check my blood pressure, pulse, and temperature. Then she'd say, "On your feet," and I dreaded that more than anything. But I also wanted to make Janet happy, and so I struggled, with help, to swing my legs over the right side of the bed. I would stand on that scale, my head bobbing back and forth, dizzy, and wait for the red numbers to show up. When they would show up, they would be in kilograms, so I never knew exactly how much my weight was falling. I only knew it was falling, but I didn't really care.

I lost, on average, eight pounds a week. This wreaked havoc with my treatments, because chemotherapy dosages are based on patient weight, and so the volume of drugs given to me was constantly being adjusted. With chemotherapy, a patient needs to have some mass, something to help it withstand the barrage, the beating, it gets from the drugs. The less one weighs, the harsher the drugs are on the body. And I had lost a great deal of mass in a short amount of time. This concerned Dr. Koufos a great deal, and he spent a lot of time encouraging me to eat, eat, eat. He even told the kitchen at the hospital to fulfill any request I had, and over the course of my seventy-day stay, I had a lot of weird requests; a head of lettuce, shredded cheddar cheese, orange sherbet, a steak.

When I dropped under 110 pounds, Dr. Koufos visited with Mom, Dad, and me and said I needed to eat nutrient-dense foods, that I especially had to eat a good breakfast to help my body deal with that day's incoming drugs.

"What do you like to drink at home," Dr. Koufos asked me.

I didn't answer, but Mom spoke up.

"He drinks iced tea," she said.

"With sugar?" Dr. Koufos asked.

"Yes," Mom said.

"Good. Get him to drink that here."

Then he said I needed to eat snacks that had a lot of calories in them. It hadn't been that long ago when I would eat a king-size Kit Kat or Reese's Peanut Butter Cup and drink a one-liter bottle of Mountain Dew every day after school, a snack that I bought with money from my part-time job at the ice cream shop in town. If I wasn't eating that, I was eating ice cream, entire pints for breakfast. None of that sounded appealing now. Mom and Dad nodded and said they would bring in other possible foods for me to eat. I did my best to ignore the conversation, as even the talk of junk food made me want to puke.

Before he left, Dr. Koufos asked me how I was doing.

"I'm tired of it all," I said, before turning my head and looking out the window.

Mom constantly gave me pep talks to keep my spirits up. She read a book titled *Love, Medicine and Miracles*, by Bernie S. Siegel, who wrote that "unconditional love is the most powerful stimulant of the immune system." Siegel was a surgeon in New Haven, Connecticut, and taught at Yale University. The book, published five years before I got sick, deals with the mindset of patients who have recently been diagnosed with cancer. The book seems kooky to me now as an adult. At one point, Siegel attributes diseases like cancer to a lack of love from one's parents; however, the entire point of the book is how much of a weapon the mind can be when fighting illness. After all, if a lack of love can cause cancer, then surely a brain fired up on love, hope, and optimism can defeat the disease.

While Mom remembers reading me passages from the book, she doesn't remember exactly what she read to me. She was constantly telling me to be positive, to be optimistic that I would go home soon, that I would be all right. At one point, she showed me a newspaper clipping of a girl who had been diagnosed with leukemia who went home from the hospital after just fourteen days. This was before I had spent two weeks in the hospital, but the point was, look, you're almost there. You're going to survive just like this girl.

At the end of a chapter titled "Disease and the Mind," Siegel writes "The patient's world may be dark, but there *are* sources of illumination. Within each of us is a spark. Call it a divine spark if you will, but it is there and can light the way to health."

Mom was trying to light a spark, and who knows, maybe she did. Maybe that is what Dr. Koufos, Theresa, and Janet all saw in me as well. But I didn't. I was resigned to a feeling of helplessness, a helplessness pervaded by thoughts that nothing mattered, including whether I lived or died. I wouldn't realize until college that I had turned into a nihilist as a childhood cancer patient, at least for a time. Sometime in those first couple of weeks, I realized, at least on the surface, that I was no longer scared of anything. I was fifteen years old and unafraid, and I was ready to die if it came to that.

Two days before Dr. Koufos practically begged me to start eating, Janet walked into my room while I was still asleep and did her normal 8 a.m. checkup. I woke up easily and noticed that she had come in with a small bag from McDonald's. In it was a sausage biscuit. I had told her three days earlier, the last time she had been my nurse, that sausage biscuits were my favorite breakfast food, and so she had stopped at the McDonald's in Orrville on her way to work because she knew how important it was that I eat something, that I fight to keep my weight (and my spirits) up. I ate the sausage biscuit sometime between noon and 1 p.m., and, fortunately, was able to hold it in my stomach the rest of the day.

Before I ate that sausage biscuit, though, I had a bath. This was just the second time I had bathed since coming to Akron Children's twelve days earlier. At 11:30 a.m., right in the middle of *The Price Is Right*, Janet unhooked the IV tubes that were running into my central line. She helped me out of bed, as she did so many times, to weigh me, to get me to sit in the chair while the sheets and blankets on the bed were changed.

"I'm dizzy," I told her.

My head was swimming. I was at an altitude I hadn't spent much time at and my brain had trouble figuring out where I was and what I was doing.

She held on to my arm as we started walking. I had to take baths because my central line could not get wet, but my room did not have a bathtub. That meant I had to walk to room 467, which was a left out of my room and then a right past the nurses' station. I was unsteady as I walked, unable to move one foot in front of the other. I felt like a toddler learning to walk for the first time. Mom was also walking with me and holding my other arm.

Once we got to the bathroom, Mom helped me undress. She peeled off my shorts and shirt, and then helped me remove my underwear. She put them in a pile to take home, to wash, and then ultimately, to bring back so I could change into them after my next bath in a week or so. I stepped, naked, into the bathtub and let the warm water fill up around me.

By now, my head didn't need to be shampooed because my hair, my precious hair, had started falling out. I woke up every morning and found thousands of brown strands attached to my pillowcase. I also frequently reached back with my left hand to twirl my hair to try and calm my nerves and ended up pulling chunks out between my fingers. Still, Mom washed my head and the few remaining hairs with a washcloth. I stood up at one point, completely naked and exposed before my mother, something no teenager would wish on anyone, and had Mom wash my legs because I couldn't bend over. Then we were done, and I dried off and put on clean clothes. Janet helped me walk back to room 462 and said that I seemed steadier on my feet now.

The bath reinvigorated me because I ate the sausage biscuit and then at 2:15 p.m., after a visit from Dr. Koufos, Dad, and I went on a walk around the nurses' station. On that walk, though, the dizziness returned, and I became unsteady. I went back to my bed, where I knew I belonged, where I figured I might never leave.

CHAPTER 5

The Fever

I woke up on a Thursday morning, just thirteen days into my stay at Akron Children's, and for once, I was hungry. It was January 17, and I had only been given one chemotherapy drug in the last three days. Additionally, the number of leukemic cells in my body was rapidly declining. When the breakfast tray came into my room, I drank the entire container of orange juice. I ate the bacon, even though it wasn't crispy like I preferred. I ate the French toast or the pancake, whatever it was that Dad had ordered for me the night before. I ate it all. Everything.

And then I threw up, but only a little bit, and it was mostly just water.

The nurse asked me if I wanted to take a bath that morning, and I said yes. I was feeling good, as good as I had since I first showed up at this hospital. The nurse helped me stand, slowly.

"How does it feel when you stand?" she asked me.

"I'm a little dizzy," I said, "but not as bad as yesterday."

After the bath, which Dad helped with, I went back to my room, and instead of climbing back into bed, I sat in the chair beside the bed. Dad and I watched *The Price Is Right* on TV, and then the noon news. I was up the whole time, either sitting in the chair or sitting up in the bed. Around noon, Dad walked to Niam's, a restaurant that was just down the street from the hospital, and got lunch. He brought me back French fries and a milkshake. I ate the fries and drank about half the shake. Then, at 2 p.m. when *Gilligan's Island* came on, Dad asked if I wanted to go for a walk around the halls. *Gilligan's Island* was by far my least favorite show during the daytime, and so I said yes. I hadn't said yes to so many questions that were focused on having me get out of bed and do something in my entire stay at the hospital. And every time I stood up, I felt better, stronger.

Whenever the nurse came into my room, and she did so five times that day, she went through the normal routine of checking my temperature, blood pressure, pulse, and respiration rate. Then she would ask me how I was feeling, if I had any pains or anything, and I told her I was fine, every time.

Mom showed up at the hospital sometime around 3 p.m. She had worked that morning at Rubbermaid, the job she had held for several years after first getting hired on through a temp agency. Mom started her working career when I was in the fourth grade, when she took a job as a waitress at a truck stop called the Chuckwagon. Now she worked in the purchasing department at the world headquarters of Rubbermaid. When I first got sick, her bosses told her to only work when she could. They put no pressure on her to show up for work, but still she wanted to be there a bit. It offered her a little normalcy. She also knew that our family's insurance was through her job, and she didn't want to risk losing that job and the insurance.

We walked around the room and the hallway for a little while. I finally climbed back into my bed a little after 3:30 p.m. and closed my eyes to rest. I was tired, but it was a good tired. I wondered when the last time I had moved around that much. Perhaps it was at basketball practice for the FFA tournament that I had, just two weeks ago, hoped I would be playing in, a tournament that had come and gone. I thought about the things I was missing. I was one of those kids who actually enjoyed going to school, who enjoyed the social interaction with everyone. And while I might have been bored in several classes and terrified of a handful of teachers, I never had trouble waking up in the morning and getting myself to the bus stop.

As I lay there, thinking about what I was missing and thinking about how good my day had been, wondering if I could be close to going back to those normal days, a faint, throbbing pain started forming in my head. If I closed my eyes, it eased a bit, but didn't go away entirely. I imagined it had something to do with all of my activitity that day, and so when the nurse came in at 4 p.m., while *DuckTales* was on the television, she asked me if I had any pain or discomfort.

"I've got a bit of a headache," I said.

She came back a few minutes later with some Tylenol, and I gulped them down.

A couple hours later, Mom asked if I felt like going for a walk again, and I said yes. She helped me up, and held my arm with one hand while she pulled the IV pole with the other. We walked slowly, but I was steadier on my feet than I had been just a few hours earlier. Outside my door and to the right, in the room next to mine, was a crib. Inside that crib was a baby, or a toddler. I could never really see inside when we walked past, and I had to rely solely on what Mom or Dad had seen on their many strolls, and even they hadn't seen much. They had seen one thing, though—or not seen something—there was never a parent in there. I couldn't imagine not having Mom or Dad with me while I was in the hospital. So far, I had spent fifteen nights in a hospital, only one of them alone, that first night in Wooster. That was the worst night. They often annoyed me when they were in the room—Dad's talking on the phone shook my nerves to no end, and the smell of Mom's microwave popcorn often made me want to throw up into the kidney-shaped bowl that sat on my bedside table.

"Get out!" I would yell at them. "I can't take it!"

Dad would go find a pay phone instead of using the phone in my room. Mom would take her popcorn to a parents' lounge around the corner from my room. Within minutes, I would pound on the nurses' call button. When the nurse would come into my room, I would tell her I needed Mom or Dad back in the room, that I couldn't take being alone.

But that baby was alone all the time, except when a nurse was in there or when a doctor was checking on him or her. And I felt for that kid. How could he or she survive?

Mom and I walked around the nurses' station and then down the hallway. We turned around after about a hundred feet, and I shuffled my feet back to my room. The walks were more like shuffles for me. The vincristine, a drug I received in two milligram doses once a week, killed the nerves in my feet, and so even though I thought I was pulling my feet up and walking normally, I wasn't. We got back to the room around 6 p.m., and the second-shift nurse walked in. I told her I still had a headache, that the Tylenol hadn't worked. At 7:30 p.m., I hit the nurses' call button and told her I needed more Tylenol, but she said it still wasn't time. I had to wait four hours after my previous dose. Finally, at 8 p.m., she came in with more Tylenol, which I gulped down again with a bottle of Gatorade that was sitting by my bed. The Tylenol seemed to help this time, and by 10, I was asleep, but not for long.

At midnight, the third-shift nurse who smelled like cigarette smoke woke me up. She needed to check my vitals, she said, and oh how I hated her when she woke me up to do these things. The sleep I was awakened from was not a deep sleep. When she started checking my blood pressure, the pain in my head flared, and this time, it was accompanied with a stomachache.

My stomach had felt kind of funny earlier in the day, but I thought nothing of it. I thought my stomach wasn't used to all the food I ate. But now, I was hit with pains up high and in my mid-section. The nurse gave me some more Tylenol just after midnight, and I fell into a light sleep. She woke me up at 4 a.m. again. This time, my stomach was throbbing and my head was pounding.

Once more with the Tylenol, and now, something for my stomach, a drug called Phenergan, which was injected directly into my central line. Because she was pushing a drug into my central line, she went ahead and took my blood, which was normally taken at 6 a.m., yet another time I would have been woken up. For this, I was thankful, thankful that I might get a little bit of uninterrupted sleep. But that was wishful thinking.

I woke up to Janet's voice at 8 a.m. There was a difference, I realized even then, about the way Janet woke me up in the morning to check my blood pressure and everything else she needed to check and the way the cigarette-smoking night nurse woke me up at midnight and 4 a.m. Janet would wake me up with a soothing voice and her soft hands on my forehead, whereas the night nurse woke me up with a gruff growl, that was followed by the smell of mentholated smoke. That smell reminded me of the days when Mom and Dad bowled in a league on Saturday nights, and my brothers and I spent hours in a bowling alley that seemed to have cigarette smoke seeping through the cracks of the walls.

Janet asked me how I was feeling, and I told her my chest and stomach hurt. I didn't mention my head. Dad had driven up to the hospital after getting John and Jim ready for school, and so both Mom and Dad helped me get out of bed after Janet left my room. As we walked around the nurses' station, I had a hard time keeping my balance. I had to hold on to someone's arm the entire time. Just sixteen hours ago, I was walking completely on my own, and now my head was swimming and my legs were weak again. Even shuffling my feet couldn't keep me from feeling like I was about to fall over. When we got back to my room, I sat in the chair. Janet came into the room and asked how I was feeling.

"Dizzy," I said.

I looked out the window toward the intersection. Outside, it was sunny and clear, one of those January days in Ohio when you look outside and think that it looks warm, but if you walk out, you get smacked by a cold wind.

I was scheduled to get a platelet transfusion at 10 that morning, and so I climbed back into my bed. Janet started that transfusion, and when she was done, she checked my vitals. When she took my temperature, I had a fever of 100.6 degrees.

A fever in a leukemia patient is just about the worst scenario one can imagine. Dr. Koufos had explained to Mom, Dad and me exactly how bad a fever could be, how white blood cells were the ones that fought infections in the body, and how just about all of my white cells were immature mutants that simply wanted to clog up my blood. They didn't want to work, and they wouldn't. To make matters worse, the chemotherapy that was being pumped into my body on a nearly daily basis had one job and one job only, and that was to kill blood cells, especially leukemic cells, but the drugs made little distinction between cells that worked and those that didn't.

I had no defense against any infection that might seep into my body, and fevers indicated infection. Invariably, Dr. Koufos had said, patients who have leukemia don't ultimately die of leukemia. Rather, he said, they end up getting some sort of bacterial infection, like pneumonia, because they have no immune system, and that is what kills them. As such, whenever anyone who spent significant amounts of time in the bacteria-rich environments of elementary schools, junior high and high schools came into my hospital room, I had to wear a mask that covered my nose and mouth. When my brothers visited on the Sunday before my central line was installed, I wore that mask as I was wheeled to the lobby, and I wore that mask when they visited me twice in my room. I wore that mask the two times my friend Pag visited, and when other friends with whom I didn't really hang out that much with at school visited. I wore that mask anytime I was wheeled anywhere in the hospital. I wore that mask all the time, and I grew to hate that mask. But that mask, Dr. Koufos said, would protect me.

But now I had a temperature and a headache that wouldn't go away. Now, it seemed, something might be wrong. The platelets infused into my body, a gift that would allow my blood to clot should I have some sort of internal bleeding. And yet, while part of me was being fixed, another part seemed to be coming apart. My head throbbed so badly I couldn't even look at the television. Eventually, Janet came in to check on me.

"How are you feeling?" she asked.

Just one day earlier, I had felt as good as I had in a very long time.

"I still have a headache," I said.

"Do you want me to get you some Tylenol?"

"No," I said. "It doesn't help."

I imagine I said it in the whiniest voice possible, a voice that was angry at the headache and angry at the Tylenol for not relieving the headache and angry at Janet for having the audacity to offer me Tylenol and angry at myself for being in the hospital in the first place, for having leukemia, for getting all these drugs and blood transfusions pumped into my body, which every day was looking less and less like the one I knew.

I had never had a headache that wouldn't go away, and this one was rumbling like a freight train through my frontal lobe. Eventually, Janet got a doctor's permission to push Demerol—the same drug I received for the bone marrow extractions—through my central line in the hope it would stop my head from pulsing and throbbing, and it did. She gave me that drug at 1 p.m., and for the next four hours, I was able to lie around, doze, and watch TV with my eyes half-closed.

While the headache went away for a few hours, the fever did not. At 4:30 p.m., it had climbed nearly a full degree, to 101.5 Fahrenheit. That was my temperature ninety minutes later. At 8:30, it had climbed again, to 101.7.

I took Tylenol for the pain, but this time, it wasn't limited to my head.

"My arms and legs ache," I said. "I'm so tired, but I can't even sleep."

"I don't feel good," I said. "I'm dizzy. I'm shaky."

Barely twenty-four hours ago, I had the best day of my two-week hospital stay. And now I felt like I was falling apart, only this time, it was worse than what sent me to the hospital in the first place, worse than any of the pains and nausea I felt because of the chemotherapy.

The lights in the hallway, fluorescent lights that never extinguished, seeped under the door to my room. The sounds of nurses walking up and down the hallway, of other sick kids' IV machines beeping, of a helicopter landing on the nearby helipad, of ambulances, sirens blaring, pulling into the emergency room below, carried into the room and into my pathetic attempts at sleep. I tossed and turned, although the tossing and the turning was hindered by my tether to an IV machine as well a machine that fed nutrients through a tube that snaked up my nose and down my throat, into my stomach. That new addition happened earlier in the day, on a Monday, when Dr. Koufos decided I was not eating enough. Over the course of the weekend, when the headaches and fever developed, I had lost nearly ten pounds. I couldn't eat anything because I was constantly nauseous, not from the chemotherapy, but from the fever, the chills, and the pain in my head.

Because of the lines that were going into my body, I could, for the most part, only lie on my back. The IV lines connected to my central line, which ran into my chest. Every movement tugged at those lines, and every tug caused the tender skin underneath the dressing to ache. So I slept on my back, and maybe occasionally on my side, but only the side that was facing the IV machine, the side that faced window and the lights of downtown Akron.

The chills created by the fever forced me to burrow deep under the covers. I already had extra blankets on the bed, and I tried to dig deep into them. I was so cold, I didn't mind the tugging of the line as I tried to get warm, and eventually I did get warm. And then, and only then, did I fall asleep for, what, thirty minutes? An hour? Despite the chills, my body, which was covered by what seemed like ten pounds of blankets, became drenched in sweat. Sweat poured off of my body and soaked through my Bugle Boy T-shirt and into the sheets, the blankets, the eggcrate foam pad that made the bed moderately comfortable, and even the mattress.

At midnight, the overnight nurse checked on me. I still had a fever. When she left, though, I bolted upright, threw the blankets off and puked into the kidney-shaped bowl. I hit the nurse's call button, and she came into my room to measure the vomit. She poured a cup of water and handed it to me.

"Drink," she said.

I put the cup to my lips, but whenever I tried to swallow, I felt the feeding tube snaking down my throat, and I started gasping for air. I thought about Theresa trying to get that tube up my nose and down my throat and into my stomach earlier in the day, how she had held a cup of water to my mouth and encouraged me to sip, sip, sip, as she pushed the tube up my nose, how I gagged and couldn't breath. She had to give up the first time because she couldn't get it into my stomach. I was fighting it so hard. She came back a second time and got the tube in, giving my body one more chance to keep from starving to death.

When the night nurse left, I floated in that state between wakefulness and sleep, that space where you can't tell if what is going through your brain is actual thinking or dreams. There were so many nights when I felt like I had just fallen asleep, only to be awakened by the screeching beeps of my IV machine, which had run dry of fluids or the chemotherapy drug that was continuously infusing. So I would punch the nurse's call light button and curse the fact that she couldn't time travel to stop the beeping before it started, to let me get just a little sleep.

So I would lie there, drenched in sweat, unable to uncover for fear of being cold, unable to stay covered for being too warm. Unable to lie on my stomach and sleep, like I used to do when I first went to bed, because that was how I could fall asleep. Unable to dream or even to think, because my brain was overwhelmed. I wanted to cry. At times I wanted to scream. I wanted to sleep, for two hours. For five hours. For a month. Forever.

CHAPTER 6

The Infection

The fevers and the headaches wouldn't go away, so Dr. Koufos put me on a series of antibiotics. Most of them were administered via IV, which meant I sometimes had chemotherapy drugs pumping in one port and an IV going into another. Fortunately, the volume of chemo was less now that I was nearly three weeks into my treatment plan. Now, we had moved on to a phase that still required drugs on a regular basis, but not nearly as many or as often.

This is the time when I should have been going home. Just like the newspaper story Mom showed me of the girl who had leukemia who went home after just two weeks in the hospital, I would have done the same if it hadn't been for the headaches followed by the fever. While Dr. Koufos was confident the antibiotics he put me on would take care of the problem, he still needed to find out exactly what the problem was.

That's how I found myself, on a Thursday morning, twenty days into my hospital stay, lying on a table in a room on the second floor of Akron Children's Hospital being told not to move at all. The top part of my body was about to be inserted into a CT machine, which looked like a giant white doughnut.

Over the course of the last week, Dr. Koufos had ordered blood cultures to see what might be causing my infection. One blood sample grew a Gram-positive coccus that was not yet identified.

"Certainly in a patient as immunocompromised as this patient," wrote Dr. Blaise L. Congeni, a physician that Dr. Koufos consulted with, "bacterial meningitis, as well as brain abscess and fungal entities and protozoan entities such as toxoplasmosis all have to be considered."

Before the CT scan, though, Dr. Koufos wanted to do a spinal tap, or a lumbar puncture to be technical. I needed to have chemotherapy injected directly into my spinal column to kill any possible leukemic cells that were growing in that fluid. Dr. Koufos also wanted to pull some of the fluid out to see if there were any bacteria there that might have led to a possible infection in my brain.

I was wheeled to an exam room for a spinal tap. I'd had a few of these during my stay in the hospital, and I hated them. Dr. Koufos gave me Demerol to help dull the pain, but even that wasn't working much anymore. I took off my T-shirt and climbed slowly onto the hard examination table. Then I lay down and curled into a fetal position, sticking my lower back out as far as I could. I put headphones over my ears, pushed play on my Walkman, and the sounds of Jon Bon Jovi's album *Blaze of Glory*, the soundtrack from the *Young Guns II* movie, started playing. I grabbed Mom's fingers with one of my hands, preparing to squeeze at the first sign of pain.

"You'll feel a little bee sting," Dr. Koufos said as he started numbing my lower back with Novacain. I squeezed Mom's fingers and willed the Demerol to kick in, to knock me out.

"A little pressure now," Dr. Koufos said, as he slid a 22-gauge, two-and-a-half inch needle, into my back, between my L3 and L4 vertebra.

I squeezed Mom's fingers. I squeezed as hard as I could and tried to float away on the music that was pushing through my Walkman, which at this point would have been a song about dying young and going down in a blaze of glory. I didn't see the irony at the time.

Mom only let me hold on to two of her fingers. That's what a nurse had told her when these spinal taps first started happening. The nurse said that if she let me hold her whole hand, I would squeeze and possibly hurt her. The same would go for four or even three fingers. But with just two fingers, I could squeeze with all of the muscles I didn't have and the pain would never be transferred from me to her, but it would make me feel better.

Dr. Koufos pulled three cc of spinal fluid out of my back, which he sent off for testing. Then he injected twelve milligrams of methotrexate, a chemotherapy drug. When he was done, he pulled the needle out and patted me on the shoulder. It had all taken less than fifteen minutes, but I had managed to zone out, to put myself into a semisleep that involved my hand, clutched as hard as possible, onto Mom's fingers. I hadn't even made it to the song "Never Say Die."

Dr. Koufos came into my room later that day with the results from the CT scan and the spinal tap. It seemed, he said, they had found the culprit of my fever. The report he got from the doctor who did the scan said, "There is a focus of white matter abnormality with diminished attenuation, but no enhancement or mass effect." But Dr. Koufos would not have just read the report to us. He wouldn't have used those words either because he wanted to make sure there was never any confusion at all as to what he was saying. He was different, we had found, all independently at that point, from the other doctors we saw, doctors who spoke in confusing, medical-professional terminology and who didn't take the time to answer questions. No, Dr. Koufos spoke like a normal person and sat on the edge of my bed answering questions.

As such, this is what he told us: I had spots on my brain, and those spots were most likely causing my fever and my headaches. He said the scan couldn't determine exactly what the white spots were, but they were not typical of an abscess (an infection on the brain). But, he said, my spinal fluid tested negative for bacteria. Because he wanted to make sure that was a correct reading, he had ordered another spinal tap. For that same day. So less than eight hours after my doctor had injected a needle the size of a straw into my lower back, we were in the same room and he was doing it again.

In his notes, Dr. Koufos says that I "tolerated procedure well," but I can't imagine that was wholly accurate. It may have been physically accurate. I may have been able to lie there, completely still, trying to crush Mom's fingers, trying to focus on Bon Jovi and his songs about dying young and how blood (relatives) can betray you. But mentally, two spinal taps and a CT scan in one day, coupled with headaches and a fever that would not go away, was doing a number on me mentally. One week earlier, I had started feeling like I might be able to go home, and now I was caught in a cycle that I couldn't get out of.

The next month was punctuated by spinal taps and CT scans, as Dr. Koufos and the other specialists at Akron Children's Hospital tried to figure out exactly what was on my brain. Two days after the initial CT scan, another one was performed, and this showed another spot, or a lesion, in the left frontal area of my brain. Dr. Koufos had kept me on several antibiotics to try and battle whatever it was that was on my brain, and while the headaches seemed to recede, the fever did not. Ten days after the second CT scan, I was sent back down to the whirring metal doughnut and told to lie completely still. I willed myself to sleep to ignore the itching of my nose and my toes and everything else that came alive in that machine.

Later that day, Dr. Koufos came in to my room with the results. I was quiet, as I had been for about the last week. My hair was now gone, with the exception of one long clump that clung to the top of my head. My eyes had sunken in. The feeding supplements had stabilized my weight, but I still looked emaciated. I could walk around but got dizzy whenever I stood up, and so I tried to avoid doing that as much as possible. I knew I needed to walk, but I hated pulling two machines—the IV and feeding pumps—around everywhere I went. I had three tubes constantly snaking into my body, two into the central line and one into my nose. I wanted time away from those pumps and those tubes more than anything else.

On January 29, Dr. Koufos noted that I was "probably depressed." Anymore, when he came into my room, I claimed sleepiness, like I just wanted to close my eyes. I didn't complain of having headaches or even of chills from my fevers. My throat had stopped hurting.

I was just tired, but I was tired of it all, most notably being stuck in this hospital room.

On Sunday morning, Dr. Koufos walked into my room at 10 a.m. I had been feeling a little better. The day before, I ate two muffins and a bowl of cereal for breakfast. Later that day, I ate a bowl of soup and crackers, and then I ate an entire small pizza.

I answered Dr. Koufos's questions and even made eye contact. My nurse that day said I seemed to be in good spirits.

"How would you like to go home for a few hours," Dr. Koufos asked me.

"Yes," I said. I wanted nothing more than to get out of the hospital.

It would just be a for a little bit, and I would have to come back that evening, Dr. Koufos said, and I would have to wear the mask all the way home. And if anyone at home was sick, I would have to wear the mask there too. I didn't care. I wanted to get out, to get away from the hospital bed, to see my house, my bedroom.

A nurse came into my room at 11 a.m. and disconnected the IV antibiotics that had been flowing into me. Then she clamped off my feeding tube. Thirty minutes later, I was in a wheelchair heading across the bridge that I had crossed thirty days earlier, the bridge that had brought me to the hospital I thought I might never leave.

Dad drove me home. It was a beautiful day. Sunny and in the low fifties. There wasn't a cloud in the sky. If I hadn't been sick, I would have spent this day outside, throwing a baseball with John, or throwing a tennis ball against the railroad ties that lined our driveway, pretending I was pitching in the major leagues.

I hadn't seen John and Jim in a while. They had visited me in the hospital, but I didn't recall them coming to my room. When they were there, I was asleep, lying in bed, bald, moaning whenever I moved just a bit. They were freaked out by how I looked, as were many people who came and visited. The last time I had seen John and Jim had been that first Sunday in the hospital, nearly a month earlier, when I was wheeled down to the lobby of the hospital and we stared silently at each other, unsure of what to say because none of us had any clue what was going on.

Grandma and Grandpa McEowen, my mom's parents, were at the house, and so was my Uncle Randy, my dad's younger brother. Randy had been driving my dad's semi for the last month to make sure we still had that income. The house smelled like a roast was in the oven. That was something Mom often made on Sundays, and it was one of my favorite meals. We sat at the table and dug into the food. I put roast beef, potatoes, and carrots on my plate, and then mashed the potatoes like I always did. I lathered the potatoes in butter, put ketchup on the roast, and then dumped massive amounts of salt over all of it. I started shoveling it into my mouth. It must have been a strange sight—someone with no hair and virtually no body mass, someone with a plastic feeding tube starting behind his ear, taped to his cheek and then heading up his nose cramming food into his mouth—but I didn't care. It was the best food I had eaten in a long time, and if I ended up puking afterward, so be it.

After we were all done eating, I walked into my bedroom. I turned on my TV, the one I had bought with my own money after getting a job during the summer between seventh and eighth grades at the Golden Bear Dariette, the local ice cream stand. I flipped through the channels and saw the Chicago Bulls were playing the Los Angeles Lakers on NBC. I left it there and climbed into my own bed. I pulled the covers up and watched the game, dozing in and out of sleep, perfectly content for the first time in a long time. I didn't want to leave this place, ever.

At 4:30 p.m., just four hours after I had gotten home, Mom came into my room.

"It's time to go back," she said.

"No!" I cried. "I don't want to go back!"

"You have to go back," Mom said. "Dr. Koufos said so."

"I hate that place!" I said, tears streaming down my face. "I want to stay."

"We can't," she said.

Eventually, I got out of bed. I said goodbye to everyone and climbed back in the van. At 5:15 p.m., I was wheeled back into my room, back to my other bed, the one I hated, the one I couldn't get away from.

Good days were always followed by bad days. On February 5, when Dr. Koufos delivered the results of my third CT scan, he said it showed significant difference. What had once just been white spots on my brain was now five distrinct, small lesions.

"These most probably represent small abscesses," Dr. Koufos said.

I had a full-blown infection on my brain.

The neurosurgeons, Dr. Koufos said, were tempted to do a biopsy— that would involve drilling a hole into my skull and taking samples of the infection—but they wanted to see if the antibiotics I was on would have an effect. He said I'd have another CT scan in a week and go from there.

After delivering all of this news, after proving that good days almost always ended badly, Dr. Koufos told me it was time for a spinal tap. And after the spinal tap, a bone marrow biopsy. Because of the need for both procedures, Dr. Koufos gave me plenty of Demerol and essentially knocked me out cold.

The next day, Dr. Koufos came into my room with the results from the bone marrow test. It appeared, he said, that nearly all of the leukemic cells were gone. I was officially in remission. The massive doses of chemotherapy in those first three weeks had done exactly what they were supposed to, and that was obliterate the cancer cells in my bone marrow (and everywhere else) as well as shock the marrow into making normal cells again. Now, for the next two years, I would continue to receive chemotherapy to make sure the mutant cells don't try to rebound. We would follow a schedule of drugs that was laid out in tiny print on a thirteen-page document. We had cleared, Dr. Koufos said, the first hurdle. It didn't mean I was cured yet, but it was good news.

"Matt feels about the same today," Dr. Benson, a resident physician who frequently saw me, wrote in my Physician's Progress Record on February 12, a Tuesday. "CT of head. Slight 1 mm englargement of lesions. No new lesions noted."

From Kenneth F. Swanson, the doctor who did my CT scan: "There is essentially no change in the appearance of the brain. Five small abscesses are again demonstrated. At most, these abscesses are 1-2 millimeters larger than on previous study of 5 February, 1991."

And then the next day from Dr. Benson: "Neurosurgery to see him today."

Miss Gochnauer, my ninth-grade English teacher, visited me on Thursday afternoon. It was Valentine's Day, and she brought with her a whole bunch of cards from my friends and other students at my high school. Earlier in the week, I had received some homemade cards from some fourth graders at my old elementary school. Among the cards from my friends, Miss G also brought with her a card with a teddy bear holding a heart on the front, which was signed by the office aides at my high school. Miss G gave me a card as well. That card had a mouse on the front that was holding onto a heart that was floating away, and on the heart was "A Valentine for My Friend."

Miss G was the only teacher that I am aware of who visited me in the hospital, and she did so multiple times. She often had my class write notes to me, and then she would bring them up to room 462 and hand-deliver them. Then she would sit and talk, with me if I was talkative, or with Mom if I wasn't. Her visits made me feel guilty because, as students, we treated her horribly. She was the one teacher in the school that students trampled over. We did whatever we wanted to do in her class, and we never got in trouble. One student took the *Romeo and Juliet* record that we had been listening to in class once and hid it, which resulted in a class of Miss G hunting for it while everyone else laughed at her. Another student in the class sat in the back and systematically pulled up tiles off the floor and then dropped and smashed them.

But she was there. She was the only one who visited, the only one who sent multiple cards, and by multiple, I mean she sent me at least eight cards during my hospital stay.

After Mom pinned the new cards to the bulletin board, Dr. Koufos walked in and brought two other doctors, neurosurgeons, with him. They shined lights in my eyes and felt my neck. They asked questions about my headaches and fevers. Ultimately, they decided they needed to biopsy whatever it was that was on my brain, and that meant they were going to drill holes in my skull.

Four days later, the surgeon walked into my room. He had copies of my latest CT scan, and, as I lay in bed, trying to ignore what was happening, he marked Xs on my head that lined up with where the infections were. As he did this, he explained what they were going to do. I would be given a general anesthetic, and he would cut open parts of my scalp, then drill through the skull. Then he would stick a needle into the infected parts and pull out some of the pus so it could be tested. He handed Mom a form that she had to sign, agreeing to the "Craniotomy for Brain Biopsy," and she signed it. He said the surgery should happen at 2 p.m. the next day. Then he left.

I was in the middle of a good day. For starters, the feeding tube had been pulled out of my nose. I had gained sixteen pounds over the course of the last week, and Dr. Koufos decided that I was eating well enough that I didn't need the nutritional supplements. I had also been feeling well, sitting up in my bed, talking to Mom, the nurses, and even Dr. Koufos when he came in.

While many pieces of news sent me spiraling into depression—news of an impending spinal tap, or of the feeding tube being replaced after the current one became clogged, or even of finding out that my television shows were being preempted by news about Desert Storm—this news, the fact that a man was going to remove parts of my skull in order to get a close look at something on my brain, this generated a little bit of excitement in me. I thought this was cool. I thought this was going to be an amazing story to tell my friends when I finally got back to school. How many people could claim to have had brain surgery, I wondered.

The fact that I was thinking about bragging about brain surgery at school meant that, at least on this day, I was actually thinking about surviving, about living. I wasn't wrapped up in a cocoon of pain, misery, and a belief that I would never leave the room. Maybe it was the fact that I had now gone home on day passes twice over the last two weeks. Dr. Koufos had let me go home two days earlier, a Saturday, because he was concerned that I was getting depressed, that I was giving up. It apparently had worked. It worked so well I was excited for brain surgery.

I woke up the next morning around 8 a.m. when a nurse came in to check my vital signs.

"How are you feeling today?" she asked me.

"I'm tired," I said. "Why can't you let me sleep in?"

The excitement was gone, replaced instead with a twisted stomach and twisted nerves.

During the night, I had been hooked up to a cardiac monitor and she checked that. She checked my lungs with her stethoscope and said they sounded clean. She checked my central line dressing and said it was dry. Then she helped me up into a wheelchair, and an orderly took me back down to the second floor for another CT scan, my fifth in the last four weeks. It didn't take long. I was back in my room in less than forty-five minutes. By 10 a.m., both Mom and Dad were in my room. Dad had finally started driving his truck again recently and had been in southwestern Ohio. He had stopped at Grandma and Grandpa McEowen's, his in-laws, and when he called Mom, she told him I was scheduled for surgery. Dad called his dispatcher and said someone needed to pick up his trailer because he was leaving it where it was parked so he could drive up to the hospital.

Then, at 11 a.m., Pastor Don showed up. The room was tense. A few weeks earlier, I had asked Mom to bring a clock up to my room because I hated not knowing what time it was. She took the clock from our main bathroom (I'm not sure why we had a clock in our bathroom), and hung it on the bulletin board in a space she cleared from all the cards. I fidgeted in my bed, staring at that clock. Shortly after Pastor Don showed up, a nurse started me on a platelets transfusion. This would be necessary because of the surgery.

The clock ticked. Then, at 11:30, after the platelets had started infusing, Dr. Koufos walked into the room. He had the results of the CT scan from earlier in the morning. He said he had consulted with the doctors in neurosurgery, and they all agreed.

"Compared to the prior examination of 2-5-91 there has been interval improvement," the report read. "Three of the smaller lesions have resolved. The two ring enhancing lesions seen in the high right parietal lobe are now smaller in size. These findings are most consistent with resolving septic emboli."

What did this mean?

"The infection is getting smaller," Dr. Koufos said. "The antibiotics appear to be working. There's no need for the surgery."

Did we cheer? Or did we all just exhale loudly? Pastor Don said a prayer, thanking God for anwering all of our prayers, for making the infections start to disappear, for saving me from brain surgery.

A nurse brought in a lunch from the hospital cafeteria at noon, and I ate half of it. Then I told Mom I really wanted Chicken McNuggets from McDonald's, and so she left to get them for me. When she returned, I ate a six-piece McNuggets and a medium fry. At 4 p.m., the afternoon nurse came into my room.

"You're very cheerful," she said.

"I'm celebrating," I told her. "No brain surgery!"

Later that evening, I sat in the chair beside my bed and played cards with Dad. Then I ate dinner—three pieces of pizza. I drank a glass of Coke and ate several pieces of garlic bread. That night, around 10 p.m., I drifted off to sleep.

The next day, Dr. Koufos came into my room and talked with Mom and Dad about sending me home. He said he wanted to get me out of the hospital, and now that it seemed we had dodged the bullet with the infection on my brain, it was time for me to go home. He said I would be discharged the next day, but I would have a nurse come to the house to continue giving me IV antibiotics until the infection on my brain was completely gone.

That day I had a nurse wheel in a TV with a Nintendo game system attached to it into the room and sat in bed and played *Bases Loaded*, a baseball game.

I slept again that night as peacefully as I had the night before. When I woke up the next morning, I was excited about going home. I ate breakfast and then lunch. Mom spent the afternoon taking all of the cards I had received off the bulletin board and putting them in a box. She packed up the flowers, the boxes of baseball cards, and the autographed photo of Bubby Brister that the Steelers quarterback had mailed me when someone told him he was my favorite player.

At 3 p.m., a nurse came into my room with instructions for Mom and Dad for when we got home. The biggest concern was, of course, a fever. If I developed a fever, I had to be taken back to the hospital, to the emergency room. Dr. Koufos came into the room and gave Mom his home phone number and his beeper number.

"Call me about anything," he said, "anytime."

At 3:50 p.m., I sat down in a wheelchair and an orderly pushed me to the elevator. We went down one floor and out into the lobby. We crossed the bridge and Mom pulled the minivan up. I climbed into the van and Mom pulled out. I was going home.

CHAPTER 7

Intensive Care

I woke up in the middle of the night. I was in my own bed, in my bedroom in our house in Apple Creek, but something wasn't right. My head was throbbing and I was shivering, and so I dug under the blankets, buried my head, and pulled my knees up to my face. I couldn't stop shivering. I don't know how long I lay like that, but at 2 a.m., Mom walked into my bedroom to check on me. I don't know what made her walk downstairs from her bedroom at that time, other than a general concern that, even though I wasn't in the hospital, someone should still be checking on me on a regular basis. I told her I was freezing cold, and that I had a headache again. Mom felt my forehead. It was on fire. She got the thermometer and stuck it in my mouth. Once it beeped, the number read 103. She immediately called Dr. Koufos at his house.

Dr. Koufos was used to calls like this, and so was his wife. It was part of the job, and it didn't take him long to shake the sleep off. Mom told him about my fever and my headache.

"Take him to the ER," Dr. Koufos said.

He would make sure I got admitted back to 4-North from there.

"We have to go back," Mom said when she hung up the phone.

"No," I cried. I couldn't go back. I wouldn't go back. I just wanted the headache and the cold to stop. We repeated the scene from my first day-trip home: Mom begging me to get up and get dressed, insisting that Dr. Koufos said I had to go back to the hospital, that I would die if I didn't. Meanwhile, I said I didn't care. I said I wanted to stay in my bed. I liked my television and the fact I had more channels to choose from than the hospital. I said I didn't feel that bad. I said I couldn't spend another day in that hospital room.

Mom won, again. By 4:15 a.m., I was back in room 462, in the bed by the window.

I had gotten to spend about thirty-six hours at home. When we went there on Thursday, I immediately took two Tylenol with codeine for the minor headache I had. After taking the pills, I zoned out on the couch in our basement, watching game shows on the USA Network. With help, I climbed up the stairs into the kitchen for dinner and then spent the rest of the night in my room, in bed, watching television.

I spent Friday just about the same way I had been living in the hospital, lying in bed and flipping through the channels on TV. I even watched the same shows. TBS showed a bunch of classic sitcoms in the early afternoon. That was the best there was to offer in the hospital, and so I spent my days there watching *I Love Lucy*, *The Andy Griffith Show*, *Gomer Pyle* and *Gilligan's Island*. Now that I was home, I had more channels to choose from, but I felt better if the shows I'd been watching for the last forty-seven days were on, like they somehow kept me safe, made me feel more comfortable.

I fell asleep more easily that night, like I did the night before, because I didn't have to worry about nurses coming in every hour and waking me up to check my vital signs. I didn't have to deal with hallway fluorescent lights bleeding into my room. But then the fever and the headache bled in instead.

The nurse took my blood pressure once I got situated in bed. It was 88 over 40. She told Dr. Koufos and Dr. Benson, both of whom would be in to see me. I was having trouble dealing with being back in the hospital, so I slid my headphones on, put Jon Bon Jovi in my Walkman, and drowned out everything around me with music blaring directly into my ears. I closed my eyes and dozed off for about an hour before being awakened so an orderly could take me to X-ray. Later that day, Dr. Koufos came in and said I needed another CT scan and then a spinal tap.

"Leave me alone," I whimpered. "I just want to sleep. Leave me alone."

They wouldn't leave me alone. My blood pressure was not increasing, and the headaches and fever were not going away. By now, a nurse was coming into my room every twenty minutes to check my blood pressure. At 1:15 p.m., it was 95 over 50. At 1:50, it was 89 over 39. Dr. Koufos and two other doctors walked into my room and talked with Dad. I stayed in bed with my headphones on, refusing to acknowledge the fact I was back in the hospital, refusing to talk to anyone.

The problem, Dr. Koufos said, was my blood pressure. It was so low, he worried I would go into shock. The fact that my heart wasn't pushing blood through my body like it should have also meant I could suffer a heart attack, a stroke, or kidney failure. I needed to be in intensive care, Dr. Koufos said, so I could be hooked up to several other monitors and have nurses and doctors keeping track of what those monitors were telling them constantly.

At 3:10 p.m., Dr. Koufos signed the order to transfer me to the ICU. Dad had told me I was being transferred to intensive care, but I didn't think anything of it. I figured it was just one more thing. I thought an orderly would show up with a wheelchair and I would be wheeled there just like I was being wheeled everywhere today. Instead, two nurses walked in, put up the handrails on my bed, and said, "Are you ready?" And before I could answer, I was being moved out of 462 in my bed.

There was no television. That was the first thing I noticed about my new room in the ICU. No television. The room was much smaller than 462, and I had no window to look out. In fact, the only windows were interior, as the walls that separated my room from the hallway and the nurses' station were glass. There was a stainless steel toilet close to my bed. I sat in bed and stared at a bunch of medical equipment that I was hooked up to now, most notably a heart monitor. I watched the green lines blip every time my heart beat. I thought of so many of the TV shows and movies I had watched where that green line represented life and death. I did not remember having been hooked up to this machine before.

When Dr. Koufos visited us the first time in the room, I told him I needed a TV, that I couldn't survive without one. He said he would see what he could do. He also said he was happy that I was alert and talking. He didn't expect that, given my blood pressure. I told him my head was hurting worse than it had in a long time, and I kept getting chills. I had already asked a nurse to bring in more blankets for my bed. My temperature hovered around 103 degrees.

Dr. Koufos said the primary goal of my stay in the ICU was to get my blood pressure up while simultaneously continuing my antibiotics for the infection on my brain. I may also need blood transfusions, he said.

"But you have to get me a TV," I said. It was all I cared about.

Before that conversation, Mom rushed back to the hospital. She had gone home after I was readmitted in the morning and had several errands to run, things that needed to be caught up with, things she had scheduled because she thought I would be home. She met Dad and Dr. Koufos in the ICU outside the glass walls of my room. If my eyes had been open, I would have seen them. But they weren't. I was sleeping, because at that moment that was all I wanted to do. I was so tired, more so now than I was even before we found out I had leukemia, back in December when I couldn't even keep my eyes open to unwrap Christmas presents at my grandparents'.

"Is he going to die?" Mom asked Dr. Koufos. She had realized on the drive back to Akron that we were not in the clear. Not even close. She had started feeling, for the first time, like she was going to lose me. Her optimism started slipping. She started to see a life without her oldest son, and she blamed herself for it. When she was climbing the stairs in the parking garage to get to the bridge, she collapsed in tears. She begged God to not take her son for her own personal shortcomings. She carried that weight across the bridge and into the ICU. It was a weight that just about everyone else carried as well, Dad, both of my brothers. Even me. We all felt like we had done something that resulted in my getting leukemia. For me, I thought God gave me leukemia because I masterbated too much. I had promised him multiple times in prayers that I wouldn't jack off anymore, but things just kept getting worse.

"Is he going to die?" Mom wanted to know as I lay in intensive care, my eyes closed, my blood pressure so low I could suffer a heart attack or kidney failure at any moment.

"I've seen sicker kids survive," Dr. Koufos said, choosing his words carefully. "But I've also seen kids not as sick not survive."

That wasn't the answer she was hoping for.

I woke up around 5 p.m. and was thirsty. I asked for a Coke and one appeared. Then a maintenance man appeared with a small television set. He moved some of the medical equipment on a shelf above my bed to the side and plopped the TV down. Then he ran some wires to the TV, handed me a remote and said, "There you go." I turned the television on and found I had all the channels I had in 462.

I drank the Coke and watched TV. A dinner tray showed up, but the food looked gross. Still, I was hungry.

"Can you get McDonald's?" I asked Mom.

"What do you want?" she asked.

"McNuggets. And fries."

An hour later, at 7 p.m., I was sitting up in bed and eating my dinner. Mom and Dad sat beside me. Dr. Koufos kept checking in every thirty minutes or so. I was feeling a little better. My heart monitor kept blipping and beeping, no flat lines yet.

I hypothesized as to why my blood pressure was so low.

"The nurses keep taking all my blood," I said, referring to the massive amounts of blood that was being drawn on my central line for all sorts of testing. They were doing regular blood counts to make sure the leukemia hadn't come back, but they were also taking large amounts of blood to test for various bacteria.

"How can I have a blood pressure," I said, "if I don't have any blood?"

It was a serious question, although Mom and Dad laughed.

"Seriously," I said. "They're like vampires!"

I drank another Coke a little after 8 p.m., and then Mom and Dad had to leave. There was no extra bed in the ICU, and they weren't allowed to spend the night anyway. They left the hospital and walked next door, to the Ronald McDonald House, which from room 462 I could see clearly, but now, not so much. That left me alone for the first time since January 2, the night I watched *Hoosiers* with a nurse in Wooster. Then, the night tears streamed down my face because I was scared, because I had no idea what was going on.

I knew what was going on now. It had been fifty-two days since that first night alone. I wasn't scared anymore. I was resigned. I didn't know what would happen, but I also didn't care, and that actually made me feel a little better. The TV flickered from its perch up near the other medical equipment. Dan Rather was reporting on Desert Storm. Then, around 10 p.m., I drifted off to sleep.

They started me on blood transfusions the next morning. Between that and the ten drugs I was given that day—Tylenol, Flagyl, Dilantin, piperacillin, nystatin, vancomycin, cefotaxime, tobramycin, Septra, and ketoconazole—my blood pressure started to recover. I spent the day watching the little television Dr. Koufos made sure I had. Nurses continued to walk into my room to check on me every fifteen to thirty minutes, and every time they walked in and asked how I was, I answered the same way.

"I feel fine," I said.

My blood pressure at 7 a.m. was 128 over 81. Three hours later it was 128 over 60. It stayed in that range all morning and early afternoon, and so at 2:30 p.m., two nurses walked into my room, put up my bed rails, and wheeled me back to 462.

CHAPTER 8

Going Home

I would spend seventeen more days in Akron Children's. Dr. Koufos wouldn't let me go this time until the infection on my brain was completely obliterated. He had let me go earlier because he saw how depressed I was getting, as well as how happy going home on a day pass made me, and he understood just how important my frame of mind was. But that had backfired when the fever came roaring back.

At home, things were getting complicated, if they already weren't. John and Jim didn't know how to process what was happening some thirty miles away in a hospital room they visited only a couple of times, and they were mortified by what they saw in those instances. Because Dad had gone back to work and Mom continued to spend the nights in the hospital with me, that meant Grandma McEowen or Grandma Bev (my dad's mother) stayed with John and Jim. We had, in many ways, grown up knowing our grandparents only in the most cursory of ways. In 1979, we had moved almost three hours away from southwestern Ohio, where both Mom's and Dad's families lived, when I was four, John was two, and Mom was pregnant with Jim. Because of that, we knew our grandparents only through annual Christmas, Thanksgiving, and other gatherings, and through the occasional one-week trip during the summer. Now John and Jim were faced with living with our grandmothers (usually just one at a time), with taking orders from them, while their brother lay in a hospital bed, dying for all they knew.

John, who was thirteen years old, snuck out at night. Jim was eleven, but was throwing fits whenever Grandma wouldn't let him do something, like stand on his drum case. The day I got out of the ICU, John told Grandma he was going to sleep in Mom and Dad's bed, but when she went to check on him, he wasn't there. She went and sat on the couch until well after midnight and waited for him. At some point, she heard the front door opening, followed by John sneaking in. He couldn't believe Grandma was sitting there waiting on him.

"Eloise came home tonight to be with the boys," Grandma McEowen wrote in her diary that night. "They are at a loss to know what to think sometimes."

I was also at a loss as to what to think. Aside from an allergic reaction to one of my chemotherapy shots on February 25, I was feeling fine. But my hospital room felt more like a jail cell than anything else, one I didn't see any way out of. Dr. Koufos made me start doing physical therapy the Thursday after I got out of the ICU, and I hated that more than I hated my hospital room. I hated how cheery the physical therapists were who came into my room to do exercises with me, and I hated the ones I met in the physical therapy room even more. They pushed and pushed and pushed, and I wanted to push back because I was so fed up with it all.

There were times at night, now that the fevers had gone away, that I was able to sleep deeply enough to dream. There is one that repeated itself a handful of times. In the dream, I was running down a hill, and after a few moments, I realized the hill was behind my elementary school, the school my brother Jim was still attending. That grassy hill was across from an alley that ran behind the school, and it led to the vast playground that we had access to as kids. To the left at the bottom of the hill was all the playground equipment—slides, merry-go-rounds, monkey bars, swings—and basketball courts. In the middle was a wide-open, big swath of grass that my friends and I used to play touch football on at recess. To the right was a baseball field, where I had played many Little League baseball games when I was younger.

The hill in the dream, though, is endless, and I keep picking up speed as I am running. At some point, I look at my left hand and see a baseball mitt on it, and inside that mitt is a baseball, and that's when I think that I'm running down for baseball practice, which makes me want to run faster.

I felt so alive in the dream, so strong and able to do whatever it is that I wanted. I didn't have leukemia in the dream or an infection on my brain. I wasn't receiving chemotherapy or antibiotics. I wasn't exhausted by physical therapy that consisted of marching in place. I was the Matt I knew before all of this started, and so I kept running and running until I woke up. I never did throw or catch a baseball in the dream, but when I woke up, I found myself yearning to be active again, to be fully alive.

Dr. Koufos let me go home on day passes on March 9 and 10—a Saturday and Sunday. Given this was the third and fourth times I had been home for a few hours, these brief visits started taking on a more routine feel. We ate big lunches together that were often my favorite foods. I cried when Mom told me it was time to go back to the hospital. I swore at her like I swore at the physical therapists. Eventually, though, I was back in the van and we were driving northeast to Akron.

Janet was my nurse the following Tuesday. When she walked into my room, I told her I was hungry but didn't want to eat anything on the breakfast tray.

"What do you want?" Janet asked.

"Cocoa Puffs and dill pickles," I said.

Janet laughed and said she would see what she could do. Because of my days when I was losing weight, Dr. Koufos had put an order into the kitchen to make sure I got whatever foods I asked for. Because of the drugs I was taking—often the prednisone mixed with one of the other chemos—my taste buds were all over the place. I asked for some weird things, but this might have been the weirdest.

A short time later, Janet walked into my room with a small box of Cocoa Puffs and two dill pickle spears on a Styrofoam tray wrapped in plastic wrap.

Like the day before, I was perfectly fine for the hours that Janet was my nurse. I went to physical therapy again, and when I got back, I sat in the chair beside my bed while my sheets were changed. I told Janet my left foot hurt, and she got me Tylenol. In the afternoon, Janet pushed me in a wheelchair to the room where Dr. Koufos did my spinal taps, and I lay through that with my headphones on and Bon Jovi playing.

But then Janet left, and I turned sour again. I told the evening nurse my foot hurt, but my tone was different. I gagged when I tried to take my pills.

"I felt fine before the spinal tap," I told the nurse at one point, after refusing to eat dinner. "Now I feel like I'm going to puke."

A Johnny Cash song flashed into my mind sometime during this last week of my stay at Akron Children's, although I don't think I knew it was Johnny Cash who was singing at the time. It was his song, "I Want To Go Home." While I didn't know any of the verses and barely knew the chorus, I had started singing it to myself and then sometimes out loud as I lay in that hospital bed and watched what had been a relatively mild winter turn into a nice spring. I thought about how much calmer my bedroom was on those days I got to go home for a few hours, compared to my hospital room, where a nurse was walking in every single hour and a doctor was coming in between those visits. I thought about the trees I would see out nine big windows in my bedroom, which originally had been built as a sunroom, how I would actually be able to feel the sun on my skin, unlike in this hospital room, where even the sunniest of days couldn't add warmth to my body.

"Let me go home," I'd sing. "Why don't you let me go home? Well I feel so homesick. I want to go home."

It was, in so many ways, the perfect thing for me to be repeating. I was different when I was at the house on those day passes. I did the same thing while I was there—ate small bits of food, lay in my bed and watched television—but the feeling of home had an effect on me. It made me feel safer than this hospital room, which, despite all of the things we had added to it—the cards on the wall, flowers, baseball cards, and clock—still felt sterile and scary.

Finally, on Wednesday, March 13, seventy days after I went into Wooster Community Hospital after nearly passing out at school, Dr. Koufos walked into room 462.

"You're going home today," he said.

PART II

OUT-PATIENT

CHAPTER 9

The Clinic

The clinic, which is what Mom and I came to call the place where I went for outpatient chemotherapy and checkups, was an antiseptic white. The only color was in the the chairs—hard plastic chairs that lined the white walls—but only in a way hard colorful chairs can be colorful, which is not very. I spent a great deal of time in the waiting room, where Mom and I would sit until an exam room came open. That space, which was essentially just an extra-wide hallway, was harsh. In our early trips, I still wanted to do nothing but lie down, like I had for so long in my hospital bed, but the chairs made that virtually impossible. I had no fat on my body, and so the hard plastic was torture on my ass, and even worse on my hips when I did try to lie down with my head in Mom's lap and the rest of me spread out. In fact, the waiting room exemplified exactly how I felt—sick and wiped out, physically and mentally, a place where comfort was impossible.

The examination rooms were not much better. They were, for the most part, typical doctors' office exam rooms that consisted of an exam table—the type that is padded plastic and covered with a strip of white paper—as well as another hard plastic chair that Mom sat in. There was a sink and there was a unit to measure blood pressure hanging on the wall, although the latter was never used because a nurse named Jackie used a machine to check my blood pressure when I arrived at the clinic. And there was a sliding pocket door that, after I would be deposited into the room by a nurse, Mom and I would stare at, waiting for Dr. Koufos to knock and slide the door open.

Between March 15, 1991, and March 8, 1993, I made seventy-five trips to Akron Children's Hospital. Eight of those involved at least one night spent in the hospital, either to receive chemotherapy or to recover from receiving chemotherapy. Those hospital stays were almost always because I was dehydrated, a by-product of the chemotherapy drugs I was still receiving. I spent fifteen nights in the hospital after my initial sixty-seven-day stay on 4-North, with the last in-patient stay happening on January 21, 1992, for hypovolemia, which is often caused by a loss of blood, a loss of blood plasma, or a loss of sodium in the bloodstream, which results in diarrhea or vomiting. According to my medical records, I was also dehydrated, which means the cause of my hypovolemia was the third possibility—lack of sodium.

Our house in Apple Creek was just about forty-two miles from Akron, which means that over the course of two years, I traveled more than 3,150 miles to a hospital to get treatments. I went to the hospital twenty-one more times through December 19, 1997, as I got checkups every six months. But it was those seventy-five trips that seared into my memory the drive, one I ended up piloting many times after I got my driver's license in November 1991.

We started out in the rolling hills outside of Apple Creek, taking a road that cut through a dozen or more Amish farms. We drove on US Route 57 through Orrville, past the Smucker's factory, and even farther, out past the industrial park where my dad had once brought us every Saturday. We hung a right on state Route 585 and continued our trek northeast, past the small town of Doylestown, where I had once envisioned playing against the Chippewa Chipps in high school basketball but, by now, knew that would never happen. Then we were out of Wayne County and on a four-lane road, Route 21, still driving through land that was mostly desolate, never much to see from the road. Once we got on Interstate 76, though, that's when it felt like we had arrived in or near the city, the big city, the place I once was so afraid of and now navigated with no trouble at all. We drove past the exit to the Rolling Acres shopping mall, where, just a year earlier, I cried and yelled at Mom because she wouldn't buy me a pair of Z. Cavaricci pants— price tag: eighty dollars—for my birthday. Then it was onto state Route 58, heading toward downtown Akron. Take the Cedar Street exit, make a right and then a left, and we were there, at the Locust Street Parking Garage, a building that was close to the intersection I used to watch out of my hospital window.

I drove through that intersection dozens of times once I had my driver's license, and I always thought about the days I watched out the window, when it was icy or snowy and cold, and cars were sliding through the intersection, unable to stop. Sometimes they crunched together, the police would come, and tow trucks would remove the vehicles. As a patient, especially during the time of the brain infection, I took pleasure in those minor wrecks. They made me feel as though someone might have been having a worse day than I was.

Once the car was parked, Mom and I walked across the third-floor bridge. I would stare to the left, because from the bridge I could see the window to room 462, and then I could see the intersection and the Ronald McDonald House, where Mom and Dad stayed when I was in intensive care. That was where they cooked so many home-cooked meals, the stuff I loved, and then walked them over to my room, desperate to get me to eat. I looked at all of that stuff, because even though I had been looking at it so regularly for a long time, this was a new view, a new angle. I could see things differently.

Prior to getting back to the exam room, I had blood drawn, had my weight taken, and had my blood pressure measured. After the blood was drawn, Jackie, an older nurse, walked into the waiting room and said, "Let's go Matt."

I stood up slowly.

"Lose the shoes and coat," she said.

I dropped my jacket on Mom and then kicked off my shoes, walked into a small room around the corner and stepped on a scale. I weighed 106.7 pounds. Then I sat in a chair as Jackie wrapped a blood pressure cuff around my thin upper arm. My blood pressure was low, 100 over 50.

My blood count was normal, but I didn't feel normal. I had been home for two days and found myself back at the hospital in an uncomfortable exam room. It didn't matter that I was going to get to leave after a few hours. It was the fact that I was back, and that I would have to keep coming back, again and again and again and again.

When Dr. Koufos slid the door open, things seemed to get better. Somehow, his simple presence in a room made me feel like I would be all right. Dr. Koufos was more than six feet tall and balding. He often wore a pair of brown dress pants and a tan dress shirt. He never wore a tie. He rarely wore a white lab coat, and never wore one when seeing his young patients because he was afraid it would scare them. He had an olive complexion and deep brown eyes.

Dr. Koufos was born in Canton, a neighboring city of Akron, in 1952, but he had only recently begun working in the hematology and oncology clinic at Akron Children's. By the time I showed up as one of his patients, Dr. Koufos had been at Akron Children's for barely two years. He had been a research scientist in Montreal, Canada, studying the various causes and potential treatments of some soft tissue cancers but had missed interacting with patients, with kids, which he had done during a fellowship at Cincinnati Children's Hospital.

Now I was one of the kids he loved to interact with, and I loved the way he talked with me.

"Hello," he said, as he walked into the exam room and moved toward the sink, where he started the water, pumped soap on his already red and chaffed hands, and started rubbing them together almost viciously. "How is everything?"

He somehow asked this question in a way that made Mom and me both think he was talking directly to us.

"I'm tired," I said.

He felt my neck for stiffness, checking for signs that the meningitis was worsening despite the heavy doses of antibiotics.

"Have you had any headaches?" he asked.

"No."

"How about bright lights. Do they bother you?"

"No."

Later that day, he would write "No meningeal signs" in my chart.

Dr. Koufos turned off the light in the room and grabbed the ophthalmoscope and shined a beam of light on the dark wall across from me.

"Focus on where that light is," he said, and then looked into my eyes. Then he asked me to follow movement with my eyes.

"No focal motor or sensory deficits," he wrote. He added that there was no swelling of my optic disc.

He told me to open my mouth and stick out my tongue, which I did.

"Good," he said.

Then he put his stethoscope into his ears, pulled the other end up to my chest, and asked me to lift my shirt.

"Sorry," he said. "This is probably cold."

He pressed it to my chest, and I took a quick gasp when the cold steel hit my chest.

"Sorry," he said."

He listened to my heart and then he listened to my lungs.

"Lungs clear," he wrote.

"Your heart sounds strong," he said so many times, and this is what has stuck with me. If I had a strong heart, then surely I would be all right. I am sure I didn't even realize he wasn't speaking metaphorically, that he was being literal. The drugs that entered my blood system through that central line all went directly to the heart, where they were then pumped throughout my body. My heart had taken a beating, was still taking a beating, and so Dr. Koufos needed to hear a heart that could still pump, that could still sustain my body. But when he said my heart was strong, I heard that I was strong, that I would be all right.

He took out a reflex hammer and tapped my knees. Nothing happened.

"NEURO – Absent DTR," he wrote. DTR stands for deep tendon reflexes. I had none.

He asked me to lie down on the table and unbutton my jeans. I did, and he felt my abdomen, all the way down to just above my pubic bone. He moved his hands from side to side, pressing deep into my pathetic body, which felt more like a bag that contained fragile bones and nothing else.

"Abdomen soft," he wrote.

After giving me a physical exam, Dr. Koufos asked Mom and me if we had any questions. I wasn't yet to the point yet where I could fathom caring about anything enough to seek more information. But as my health improved, my questions invariably centered on what I was allowed to do. Could I play in a church basketball tournament? What should I do to protect my central line if I was allowed to play in a basketball tournament? Could I play baseball? Could I spend the night at a friend's house? Could I get my ear pierced?

Mom's questions were often practical in nature. She asked about my upcoming treatments, but not before she pulled the thirteen-page treatment protocol, which she had photocopied, out of her daily planner. She asked about certain dates and certain drugs. She asked about whether I would need to be admitted for treatment, and if not, how long it would take for the chemotherapy to infuse through my central line.

Not long after that first clinic visit, Dr. Koufos had also asked Mom if she would be willing and able to administer chemotherapy to me at home. I was coming up on a treatment that would require five days of continuous infusion, and Dr. Koufos did not want me back in the hospital, given how depressed I got when I was there. Mom was willing to do whatever it took to keep me out of the hospital, and so she agreed. This was a move that resulted in a reprimand for Dr. Koufos by his superiors, as well as a home health nurse showing up at our house in Apple Creek in the morning to make sure everything was all right. But it was Mom who did most of the work, changing the bags of chemo and flushing out my central line each day. She was, for that week, my Janet or Theresa.

So if we were near that time, Mom would have asked Dr. Koufos several questions about what to do if something went wrong, and then she would get into specifics. And Dr. Koufos's answer was always the same.

"Call me."

No matter what time. No matter how small you think the problem is.

"Call me," he said.

At home, Mom took to checking my blood pressure, temperature, and pulse on a regular basis. Every four days, I lay down either on my bed or a couch, and Mom crouched beside me and began the process of changing the dressing around my central line—gently tugging and pulling the tape away, removing the gauze, wiping the entry with betadine and then alcohol swabs, laying new gauze on the site, and then taping it tightly to my chest.

I spent most of my time in my bedroom, in my bed, watching television. Occasionally, I would get out of bed and walk over to the exercise bike that Grandma and Grandpa McEowen brought up from their house in southwest Ohio. They had gotten that exercise bike years earlier, when my Grandpa has slipped on the ice and blew out his knees. He used it to rehab back then, and now I saw it as my tool for rehabilitation. It was much more pleasant to do without a perky physical therapist standing over me and encouraging me to just keep going. I would get on the bike and ride for two minutes, then three minutes, and eventually, I could keep pedaling on that thing for five minutes without getting winded. Sometimes, I would walk outside and throw a tennis ball against the concrete retaining wall outside my bedroom window, and then try and catch the rebound with my baseball mitt.

I didn't go back to school because I still couldn't focus on anything for more than a minute or two. Reading, one of my favorite things to do before going into the hospital, had become impossible. My brain couldn't focus, couldn't follow sentence to sentence. I was exhausted after just walking from my bedroom into the kitchen, which was about thirty feet. I would never have been able to survive a day at school.

Mom did have to go back to work, though. She didn't want to leave me home alone, and I didn't like the thought of isolation, so Grandma McEowen stayed with us for a while. Occasionally, if she couldn't be there, Pastor Don would come and visit with me for several hours. I didn't really talk with my Grandma much but just took comfort in knowing she was there. I have no idea what Pastor Don and I talked about in those moments, other than I imagine he filled me in on what was happening in the youth group at church.

My brothers, John and Jim, would come home after school, although I have no idea what, if anything, we did together, just as I don't remember anything about their visits to the hospital, other than they visited. John was in the eighth grade, Jim the fifth. Sometime in May, Jim was in the elementary school's production of *The Little Mermaid*, and so I went with Mom, Dad, and John. Our elementary school always put on great plays, and they were performed in the high school gym. When I was in kindergarten, I was somehow chosen to play Joseph in a Christmas musical. Later, I was the backup Cowardly Lion in *The Wizard of Oz*. John had once been a Christmas robot. I don't know what Jim was in this play. The only thing I remember about this outing—which was really my first official public outing since getting out of the hospital two months earlier—was that someone in the chorus threw up on the risers. I saw the commotion, and then I smelled the smell.

"That's puke," I told whomever I was sitting next to. I knew what puke smelled like, I said, because I had puked more than everyone else in that gym combined over the last five months.

In those early days, I hated everything about Akron Children's. The sixty-seven straight days I spent there destroyed me, both mentally and physically, and I couldn't stomach the thought of the place, let alone having to go there, even on an outpatient basis. The only thing that made it tolerable was the fact I knew I would see Dr. Koufos, and then later, as I got to know nurses like Pam and Char, I looked forward to seeing them as well. But on days when an L-asparaginase shot in the thigh or a spinal tap were scheduled, I fought Mom hard about leaving the house and going to the hospital, especially when we were making the trips twice a week. I always gave in, though, because of Dr. Koufos, and because I wanted him to see me getting better, to know that his hard work was paying off.

I loved how he talked directly to me and not necessarily to my parents, like some doctors did, like Dr. Cebul did when he asked me to leave his office so he could tell my mom that he wanted me to go to the hospital for tests. Dr. Koufos talked directly to me and told the truth, no matter how difficult it may be. I imagine the more difficult of those conversations happened with my parents when I was still in the hospital and I was semiconscious. But even in the clinic, he let me know what I needed to do to avoid getting an infection, and he told me what would happen if I didn't follow his directions.

He occasionally joked around too, although his sense of humor was incredibly dry. That was something the nurses, both on 4-North and in the clinic, loved about him, given that the older doctors who treated kids with cancer were stiff, stodgy, and often severe. Once, Dr. Koufos brought a bagel and coffee onto 4-North, set it down at the nurses's station, and then went to check on a patient. There was one nurse on the floor who would not allow food or drink at the nurses' station, and so she threw his breakfast in a trash can. The next day, Dr. Koufos brought in a coffee and a bagel and set it down in exactly the same place, and the nurse threw them away again. They continued this dance again and again and again. Theresa asked him once why he did it, and he chuckled.

"It's fun," he said.

The more I went to clinic, the more I saw the fun side of Dr. Koufos, and my hatred of having to make that drive from Apple Creek to Akron lessened. By September 1991, I was ready to return to school. I was starting out as a freshman again, taking all of the classes I had taken for exactly half the year before. I missed school often in that first year back, mainly for trips to clinic, and in those visits, I would tell him I was nervous about a test or an assignment that was coming up. That was when he would chuckle and tell me that everything would be fine.

"I almost didn't get into college," he said multiple times. "I was just going to bag groceries the rest of my life."

This story wasn't entirely true, but it was one that he told to many patients and nurses. When Dr. Koufos was in high school, back when he was just Alex, he bagged groceries at Fishers Foods in Canton, and he saved the money he earned to help pay for college, something that was an absolute certainty for a smart young man. I came to appreciate his joke or tiny white lie even more once I learned that information because I saw a doctor making fun of himself to put a patient at ease.

It was in these interactions, inside this tiny white, sterile exam room, that I felt like I came to know Dr. Koufos, at least as a fifteen-year-old. He was unlike any doctor I had ever seen. He was a man that a sick young boy could joke with if he was feeling up to it, as well as a man the same sick young boy could tell just about anything to, especially when it came to how it felt to be a sick young boy. I was already seeing him as the man who would save my life.

After Dr. Koufos completed his physical examination of me, and after he had answered whatever questions Mom had at that time, he would head out to check on other patients. Then the nurses would come in and administer whatever drug I was due to get that day. Sometimes it was a shot of L-asparaginase directly into my thigh or a chemo drug dripped into my central line. Sometimes it was a continuous infusion of daunomycin or cytosine arabinoside. Some days I received methotrexate through an IV, but it had to be infused over four hours. Those days were long and boring, but better than the days I received methotrexate via a spinal tap.

When it was all done, Dr. Koufos eventually slid his way back into the exam room and let us know the specifics of my blood tests—what my white count was and how my platelets were doing. He told us what was scheduled for my next visit, which early on could have been in two or three days. On this first visit, he told us I had a CT scan scheduled to check the infection on my brain in one week, and that I had to come back in three days for an infusion of Cytoxan.

Mom often asked about the blood results and what, exactly, all of those numbers meant. In the earliest visits, when I was still very sick, it was the white count we were most concerned with, as that number determined what I could and couldn't do, socially speaking. If the white count was too low, I had to wear the mask everywhere. The mask, coupled with my bald head and sunken-in eyes and cheek bones, made me look like death, and so I hated it. I felt as if it identified me as a dead boy walking, although in March and April, I looked like that without the mask too.

After he answered all of Mom's blood count—related questions, he told us we could head home.

"Call me if a fever develops," he said that first day in clinic, and on just about every visit after that, like it was his way of saying good-bye.

CHAPTER 10

Road to Remission

I was back in a hospital bed in late April at Akron Children's Hospital, but this time, it didn't seem too bad. I wasn't in room 462, which annoyed me slightly; rather, I was in a room around the corner, on the hallway I used to shuffle my feet along whenever Mom, Dad, a nurse, or a physical therapist insisted I get out of bed and go for a walk.

What made this visit more tolerable was the fact that I knew exactly when I would be leaving. This was part of scheduled chemotherapy, and while it was severe enough that Dr. Koufos wouldn't let Mom do it at home, I took comfort in knowing that I would be leaving in three days. And I wasn't feeling that badly. I had recovered mostly from the ten days of cranial radiation I received earlier in the month, something that had left me exhausted and dehydrated. But I was bouncing back from those things far more quickly now that I was home.

On one of the three days back in the hospital, I was in bed when Nancy Carst walked into my room. Nancy was the first person I had met at Akron Children's when I first became a resident, which now was almost four months in the past. At the time, she had been assigned as my social worker, and so she came in on that first morning and asked Mom, Dad, and me all sorts of questions about our family life. I told her I loved baseball, and she asked me who my favorite team was. She assumed, since we were in northeast Ohio, that it would be the Cleveland Indians, but I surprised her and said it was the Chicago Cubs. She said the Cubs were also her favorite team.

Nancy was always one of my favorite people to see in the hospital. She had such a soft voice and laughed whenever I said something I thought was funny, even though it usually wasn't. So I was happy to see Nancy walk in on this day.

Some of the other kids on the floor are making a game, she said. A patient named Tim had the idea because he wanted to help newly diagnosed children and their families learn about having cancer, what it will be like for them as they start treatments.

"Do you want to help," she asked.

"What do I have to do?" I said.

She handed me some index cards and a marker.

"Just write down examples of good things you've experienced here and bad things," she said.

For example, she said, write about a time a medical procedure had been postponed and that made you feel happy. Or write about throwing up. Keep it short, she said. Just mention the good and the bad things. The game, she said, was going to be a square board with spaces all around it. The good cards I wrote would move players forward. The bad cards would move them backward. Players played the game until they reached the end, which was labeled "Remission."

"It's called *Road to Remission*," Nancy said.

I told her I would help.

I started writing on the cards. I wrote about night nurses waking you up to check vitals, about getting fevers and being rushed back to the hospital. I wrote about spinal taps and bone marrow aspirations. I wrote about puking and allergic reactions to medicine. I wrote a lot of cards that would move players backward, but Mom, ever the optimist, convinced me to write about some of the good things. So I wrote about having water fights with nurses with syringes and having a brain surgery canceled at the last minute. I wrote about eating a meal and not puking it up. I wrote about going home on day passes. Eventually, I filled up all of the cards that Nancy had given me.

Not long after that stay in the hospital, Nancy started a support group for teenagers who had cancer. We met about once a month, in a room on the fourth floor. This room was the one that Mom and Dad went to when I got annoyed with them when I was a resident of 4-North. Before the meetings, Nancy spread out some snacks and drinks, and then we settled onto the chairs and couches. I don't know how many times we met. Most of the kids who were there had written cards for the board game, which means most of us were still in the thick of treatment. We would sit around and talk about our lives, how they had changed, and how we navigated this new reality. Laura Jo and Shelby sat together on one side of the room. Not long before this group started, I had seen Shelby in the waiting room of the clinic, and I couldn't help staring at her. I wasn't staring at her because she was sick, though. I was staring at her because I thought she was beautiful. She wore a wig because she had no hair, and she was as skinny as I was. I was drawn to her. Because I was an awkward fifteen-year-old, I didn't say anything to her.

Todd, who was missing his left leg because of osteogenic sarcoma, sat on the couch opposite me. He'd had probably one of the toughest lives of anyone in the support group. His left leg was amputated above the knee when he was nine years old. Then cancer came back in his right shoulder when he was eleven, his right lung when he was thirteen, his right rib when he was fourteen, and now, as he sat in this support group, it had showed up in his right knee.

One time Terri was wheeled into the room in her hospital bed. Terri was a younger girl, twelve or thirteen, who was from Millersburg, a small town close to where I lived. She looked really ill, but then again, so did I and many of the other kids. Mom had struck up a friendship with Terri's mom. Most of the patients I came to know were from suburbs of Cleveland. So when we met anyone from a town closer to us, someone from the rural areas of northeast Ohio, someone who went to a school that frequently played my school in sports, we made closer connections. Mom and Terri's mom, her name is Helen, spoke several times in the room we were talking in now, the room Terri was being wheeled into that one time.

There was a boy named Curt. He was my age, another really skinny kid who loved basketball and ached to play again. And there was Tim, the boy who came up with the idea for the board game. He had been diagnosed with a rare form of cancer called clear-cell sarcoma, which showed up as a tumor on his kidney. A week after surgeons removed that tumor, a second one was spotted, and so he underwent another surgery. Then he underwent significant amounts of chemotherapy. He talked once about going out for the swim team, and this is when I started thinking about playing baseball again. I realized that the summer of 1991 would the first time in eight years that I didn't play on a baseball team, that I didn't get to field ground balls on the infield or chase down long fly balls in the outfield, the first time I didn't get to dig into the batter's box and stare down a pitcher, send his pitch into a gap in the outfield and end up on third base with a triple.

As a group, we were a collection of kids who had been forced to grow up far earlier than we ever expected. We all had—were still—facing the possibility of death. But we didn't really want to talk about that. We didn't want to talk about mortality, to acknowledge what we all feared. Instead, we talked about how to be normal teenagers again. Laura Jo talked about going to prom. The guys, myself included, talked about sports and wondering if girls would ever like us. We talked about our classes in school, about what it was like to be bald, about any teachers we had who were not sympathetic to our plight. We talked about the nurses we loved—for me that was Janet and Theresa—and the nurses that we didn't. We talked about the things we missed at school, about how our friends responded to our illnesses.

My friends had been great. They visited me on some of my sickest days, and they carry with them an image of a friend who was slipping away. My friend Pag said he and his dad, who was my baseball coach, were once stopped by a doctor before entering my room.

"You might want to consider saying your goodbyes to him," this doctor said. I don't think that Dr. Koufos would have said this, but it could have been any of the other dozens of doctors who came in and out of my room on a regular basis. Pag has carried this, along with the image of my emaciated body, sleeping but barely breathing, around with him ever since.

We talked about siblings and parents and life, and how to live it like we had lived it before we got sick. For so long, the fight to be normal again was the one thing I focused on. I wasted a lot of time, a lot of years, trying to be the Matt from before I was sick, rather than embracing the Matt I was after. I wish someone would have come into that support group, just once, and told us that we were never going to be normal again. We had all been through an ordeal that fundamentally changed who we were as people. There was no going back. You cannot stare death in the face, especially when you are a teenager with an ingrained feeling of invincibility, and ultimately wipe that away like it never happened. Everything takes on a different significance after you walk through that fire. There was no going back. Ever. But we talked like there might be a way, like that was how we would know when we were better. It's how we tried to make sense of our worlds, places that had been turned upside down. It was too much, too heavy, for us to know that everything could disappear in an instant. We knew that plans to play in a basketball tournament could be derailed, that going to the prom might not happen. We knew that what we had now might not be there tomorrow. We knew that life was unfair, and was often too short. We knew we were mortal. We knew we might die, and, for the most part, we had come to terms with that. We knew all of this and desperately tried to forget that we knew it. Nobody came out and said that, though. Not even the longer-term survivors who sometimes showed up at the meetings, people who could tell us what life would be like in another four or five years, once we were in college or working, once we had steady boyfriends or girlfriends, once we thought we were normal again.

I'll tell you the moment I thought I was normal again.

It was a cold and blustery day in late March or early April 1992, a full year after I had written all of those cards for the game *Road to Remission* from a hospital bed at Akron Children's Hospital. I was on the Waynedale junior varsity baseball team. Coach Les Sauer had put me on the team despite the fact I still couldn't run very well. Because I couldn't run very well, I also had a hard time playing in the field. But I had gone out for the team and showed I could still hit the ball—not with any power, of course—but I made contact, I put the ball in play.

I didn't play very often. I got an at-bat every couple games, in the late innings when the contest had already been decided (and in these games, it was already decided in our favor, because we were good). One day, we were playing at Norwayne, a school that was a good thirty-five minutes by bus away from Apple Creek. In the fifth or the sixth inning, the JV coach looked at me and told me to grab a bat and a helmet, that I was going to hit.

I plopped a helmet on my head, and it rattled around, loose. We didn't have any helmets on the team that would fit the shrunken, bald head of a cancer patient. My hair had not yet grown back in because I was still getting heavy doses of chemo every couple months to keep the leukemic cells at bay, and so, with a loose helmet on my head, I grabbed a bat and walked to the on-deck circle. I timed the pitcher up. He was chubby and had long brown hair flowing out of his hat, the kind of hair I used to have. The hitter in front of me singled, and I walked to the batters' box, dug in, and stared down the pitcher.

Somehow, my ability to hit a baseball did not disappear along with my hair. Once I was strong enough in the fall of 1991, I had started going to batting cages and hitting. Then in December, during a church youth lock-in at an indoor sports facility in a neighboring town, I won a hitting contest that more than a hundred kids participated in. In the contest, we got twenty pitches in the batting cage, and we got various points for hitting the ball to different spots in the cage. I didn't miss a single pitch. When I climbed out of the cage and pulled the helmet off my head, mouths dropped.

I carried that confidence with me to home plate in this at-bat. As I stood there, I forgot that I had a central line taped to my chest and wrapped in an Ace bandage. I forgot that I had chemotherapy scheduled in a couple weeks. I felt exactly like I did in that batting cage, or when I was the starting shortstop and number three hitter on my fourteen-and-under team in the summer of 1990.

I watched a couple of pitches go by. A strike. A ball. Then the chubby kid with my long, flowing brown hair delivered a pitch and I swung and shot the ball back up the middle, past the pitcher, between the second baseman and shortstop. The centerfielder raced in to the ball as I was still running to first. My friend Jamie Walters was coaching first base. He had christened me Slo Mo that season, because he said it looked like I was always running in slow motion. I pushed with every ounce of diminished muscle in my legs. The helmet bobbled on my head. And when my foot hit first base, I realized the centerfielder had just tossed the ball to second. I had my first postcancer hit. I was normal again.

Or so I thought.

Sometime just before that base hit, before I had gotten back to the world of baseball that I loved so much, I was given a board game on a trip to clinic. It was the official *Road to Remission*. The box was colorful—bright pink and blue sides; big yellow block letters; and blues, greens and oranges all over the box like confetti falling, a ticker-tape parade for the kid who has made it to remission. Along the bottom right of the box, big blue letters state that the game is "Kid Tested!" Below that are eight names, including my own, along with Tim Snyder, Todd Seitz, Terri Morris, John Lamb, Laura Jo Mounsey, Shelby Lieb, and Michael Gray.

I opened the box and looked at the board. It was the same explosion of colors as the box itself. There were picture of syringes and stethoscopes on the board too, but in a way that looks fun.

There were about seventy-five cards that came with the game, along with a bunch of blank cards so kids and parents could write their own situations on them. The first time I looked through those cards, I searched for the ones I might have written or the ones that were similar to something I had written.

"You're sleeping and the nurse wakes you up to give you a sleeping pill."
"IV beeps all through the night."
"Your feeding tube gets clogged up."
"You get a sore throat from the feeding tube."
"Chemo gives you mouth sores."

"Nothing on hospital TV."

It wasn't all negative, though. I did write things that let a player move forward.

"Your parents bring your favorite food."

"You have a water fight with the nurses and you win!"

"You get to go home on a day pass."

We never played the game at home, though. It went straight onto the shelves in our basement and sat there for several years, before I moved into my first apartment after college, and by then, so much had changed, including the idea that somehow remission was the ultimate end of the road, that the game ended there. For too many, it didn't.

CHAPTER 11

Camp CHOPS

On the second weekend in June, at the tail end of my first spring as a cancer patient, I went back to Akron Children's for a clinic visit. After going through the typical routine, I went downstairs to the auditorium where it seemed like hundreds of patients from the clinic, both current and former, gathered for Camp CHOPS. The acronym CHOPS stands for Children's Hematology and Oncology Patients and Staff. The counselors at the camp were all employees of the clinic or family members of employees. There were nurses at the camp the entire weekend, and the doctors tended to drop in for visits. Most of the patients were kids who had long since recovered from their illnesses. Those who were too sick or were still in the hospital didn't go. That June, I was one of the sickest out of all the kids there. There had been intense discussions between doctors and nurses in the clinic as to whether I should go or not. Ultimately, they took a chance. Dr. Koufos thought that I looked well enough during my clinic visit, so they put me on the bus and I rode from the hospital to Camp Christopher in Bath.

The campground was owned by a local Catholic diocese, and as such, there was a statue of the Virgin Mary on the far side of the pond that kids paddled canoes on. For this weekend, the campground was overrun with kids who had no hair or kids who were thin, kids who needed frequent medication, and kids who had at one time or another faced the possibility of death, whether they knew it or not.

We got there on Friday afternoon after a bus ride that included Theresa passing us in her Pontiac LeMans. Todd had ridden with Theresa because he didn't want to ride the bus. Then, in the car, he begged Theresa to pass the bus while we were on the interstate. When she did, he took off his artificial leg and stuck it up through her open sunroof and waved it at those of us on the bus. We lost it, collectively, and started yelling and screaming and cheering. I could see Todd in the car, his mouth open, laughing, as he held on to his leg with two hands and kept shaking it at us.

We spent two nights at the camp in cabins. It reminded me of the church camps I had gone to so many times, a church camp I would have been going to that summer had I not gotten sick, a church camp my brother John would go to and be peppered with questions as to where I was. Camp CHOPS wasn't so different, aside from the fact it only took place on the weekend and the only prayers being said were likely by parents who had sent their sick children off to camp, prayers that something wouldn't happen, that a central line wouldn't get ripped out or a sick body become infected.

On Friday night, Curt and I stayed in our cabin instead of heading down to the dining hall to make ice cream sundaes. We shared a bunk bed, with Curt taking the top and me the bottom. He had brought a boom box, and he tuned it to an AM radio station that had the third game of the NBA Finals on. I had become a Chicago Bulls fan as Michael Jordan started his rise to stardom, as had Curt. Just about every teenage boy in the early 1990s loved the Bulls, and so we lay on our bunks and pulled for Chicago to beat the Lakers. Game three was being played about twenty-four hundred miles away in Los Angeles, but we listened to the game like we were there, like we were part of the Bulls. The fact that we were spending a night at summer camp in much the same way we had spent so many days in the hospital—just lying in bed—never really occurred to us. It was such a different atmosphere, one in which we felt free to do what we wanted. The beds were comfortable despite the fact they were thin and cheap. The sounds of the announcers and of squeaking sneakers that courtside microphones picked up was infinitely more comforting than the sounds of nurses' shoes squeaking on tile floors, of IV machines bleeting out.

At halftime, we walked up to the dining hall to get ice cream and check in with our counselors, but then we went straight back to the cabin. A nurse checked in on us once or twice, but we were fine. The Bulls won the game in overtime, and Curt and I high-fived each other. Michael Jordan scored a game-high twenty-nine points and had nine assists. The game would give the Bulls the momentum they needed to go on and win the series, four games to one. It felt good to feel like a winner for the first time in a long time.

The next afternoon, while the other kids were swimming or canoeing or playing basketball on the courts up by the dining hall, I sat on the aluminum dock that jutted out into the pond. I wasn't ready yet to try to play basketball. I didn't have the energy or the strength to get the ball up to the hoop. I couldn't swim because of my central line, and I didn't want to go out in a canoe because I was afraid I would somehow capsize and get my central line wet. So I hung out on the dock.

It was sunny and warm—the temperature reaching into the 80s—but I was cold. I wore my Chicago Cubs jacket and a Cubs hat. I pulled my shoes off my feet and dipped them in the water. I had headphones over my ears and the Walkman tuned to an AM radio station, which was broadcasting a baseball game. I longed for baseball that summer more than ever, so I took it in every way possible. I wore the clothes. I listened to games. I dreamed of when I might play again, while also thinking I would never play again.

I sat on the dock in a trance. I was mesmerized by the sun bouncing off the water, by the water lapping at my toes, by the sounds of the game I loved bouncing around in my ears, by the views of kids playing in sand or paddling canoes. There was so much happening around me, chaos and order, all thrown together on one pond and beach, and it all filtered in to me in the most serene way. I could have sat there for hours, for days, for weeks. It was the first time in eight months that I felt good, right. I warmed up, and took off my jacket, lay back on the warm aluminum, and let the sun pound down on me.

There was a dance on Saturday night, and I hung out on the sides, sitting on wooden benches that lined the main activity center of the camp, and watched a bunch of kids and their nurses dance to songs like Mariah Carey's "I Don't Wanna Cry," Extreme's "More Than Words," and Roxette's "Joyride," which I thought was the best song of all. I ate pizza when they brought it, and eventually was pulled out onto the dance floor by Theresa or another one of the nurses. There was so much laughing. It was the most normal thing I had done in a very long time.

The next day, after we ate lunch, we all went to a grassy area near the front of the camp. Our parents started arriving, but before we went home, our counselors all gave us a cheesy award, a certificate to recognize something unique about us. Curt and I both received basketball-related honors, not for playing of course, but for our steadfast refusal to join an ice cream social because the Bulls' game was on.

After that, we all went home.

I met Melissa at Camp CHOPS the following June. Like me, she had been a first-time camper the year before. But I had spent so much time in the cabin listening to basketball and the rest of the time wandering around the camp by myself that we didn't interact.

Melissa was nineteen years old when she came back to Camp CHOPS in June 1992. She realized something wasn't right within her body in October 1990, just a month before my bone marrow started spewing out leukemic cells. She was suffering from severe abdominal pains. She went to the doctor, and found out she had rhabdomyosarcoma. Within a day or two, she was under the knife, a seventeen-year-old having a complete hysterectomy. From there, she was sent to Akron Children's Hospital to start chemo. This was during her senior year. She had been such a good student for the first three years of high school that she needed just one more credit to graduate. The school district gave it to her, and she graduated with her friends. She could barely walk across the stage because the chemotherapy had deadened her feet and legs.

Dr. Koufos took care of her for the couple of months she spent in the hospital receiving chemotherapy. She was back home by the time I showed up, so we never crossed paths in the hospital. Our diseases were incredibly different, although the effects on our bodies were about the same. In June 1992, when we finally met and talked to each other about our cancers, we were both in the process of getting better.

She was planning on going to college in the fall after having taken a year off from school to recover. She hadn't been in school since she got sick eighteen months earlier. I had just finished my first complete year of high school, having restarted as a freshman. Because I hadn't gone back to school after going into the hospital, and had done no work at home, I had just half-a-credit to my name, for typing class. I had also just finished my first season as a high school baseball player and had gotten several hits as a bench warmer on the junior varsity team.

We were no longer campers at Camp CHOPS because we were both over sixteen and had at least one year of experience as a camper. We were now counselors-in-training, or CITs as we became known around camp, and we had to work. There were six CITs that weekend. Todd was one, and along with Melissa and me, we were the three that were still undergoing treatments for our various cancers. The other three were Ben—the son of my clinic nurse Pam and a boy my age who shared many of the same interests as me—and Sharon and Kim, both teenage girls who survived their cancers when they were younger. As CITs, we found ourselves doing all the grunt work at camp. We filled water bottles and made snow cones and helped the regular counselors however we could by watching campers or taking little kids out on the pond, something I was exempt from because of my central line. We helped usher the younger kids through the food lines and took others to the bathroom. When we didn't have anything to do that was pressing, though, we just hung out.

Like the previous year, I spent some time lying in my bunk, listening to Ben's Eric Clapton cassettes. At one point, on Saturday, we took a hayride, and I sat beside Melissa. We talked about the various things we cancer patients had to go through: the weird stares from strangers, how our friendships were different now, how we could pretty much say or do anything we wanted without getting in trouble.

We also talked about the way we walked now.

"The stork walk," Melissa called it.

One of the chemotherapy drugs we both took—vincristine—killed the nerves in our feet. This caused us to shuffle as we walked, rather than actually picking our feet up and stepping like normal people. Shuffling, of course, led to tripping on the slightest cracks in sidewalks or floors. That happened to me on the one day I went back to my high school for a half-day of classes, mostly to visit with people and let them know that I was still alive. On that day, Pag, Doug, and I were walking from the high school to the junior high building, where we had vocational agriculture, and I tripped on the sidewalk. I went down hard, but scrambled back up like nothing had happened. We walked the rest of the way to class, but when I sat down, my friends noticed the red seeping through my stonewashed jeans. I had peeled away the fragile skin from my left knee. I shoved hard, brown paper towels up my jeans, onto my knee, and told everyone it was fine, that I was all right.

To combat these missteps we deliberately picked our legs up high and took incredibly careful steps. And because our legs were so skinny, we looked like storks. I laughed at Melissa's dubbing of the stork walk. I loved how she could say things that seemed to be on my brain as well, things that I thought about but never really let leave my head. Melissa had no trouble letting loose the thoughts that floated in her brain, and she verbalized those thoughts in a loud, brassy voice that made her sound like she had come to Camp CHOPS straight from Boston.

On Friday night, Ben, Sharon, Melissa, and I crowded into the basket of a hot-air balloon that was tethered to the ground. The camp had planned to let kids go up and then come right back down, but it was too windy. So we stood in the basket and posed for a picture. I stood next to Melissa, and while I didn't know her as well as I would come to in the next year, I was still sixteen years old and enjoyed standing so close to a girl, a woman actually, that we actually touched. The balloon was the colors of the rainbow, and it looked like it wanted to float away. I thought that would be amazing if we all found ourselves lifted up and away, away from everything we had been going through over the last year or so.

We stood for the camera, and everyone except for Ben was stone-faced, flat-mouthed, a dead stare pushing outward. Our facial expressions resembled those of people from photographs in the late nineteenth and early twentieth centuries, when they thought smiling made them look silly. I felt my thinness standing next to Ben, who was wearing a T-shirt with the sleeves cut off, huge arms protruding out. I wore a Chicago Cubs T-shirt that Pag's mom made for my sixteenth birthday, and Melissa wore a maroon T-shirt with the sleeves rolled up. Sharon stood in the back, on her tiptoes so her face could peer out between the other bodies. Ben had a hat on backward and beamed a huge smile.

A photographer hit the button on the camera and our image was sealed forever on film.

Todd 's left leg was amputated above the knee when he was nine years old. That was seven years before I met him in our support group meetings, eight years before we all gathered at Camp CHOPS as counselors-in-training.

It's hard to describe Todd in any way other than to say he was bald (like so many of us) and maybe he was borderline crazy while simultaneously being the life of the party. He found humor in everything, including losing a leg at the age of nine. That was when he told the surgeon to go ahead and amputate both legs. That way, he could be as tall as he wanted thanks to prosthetics.

That Saturday, we got a break from our CIT duties, so we walked up to the stables at the camp. I was nervous because I had never been on a horse, at least not unsupervised. But Kim had spent her life around horses, and she said we would all be fine. And by this time, I wasn't about to not do something Melissa was doing.

After a short instruction on how to ride, we all got our horses and mounted them. Kim, Sharon, Ben, and Melissa took off through the woods like they had all been riding forever. Todd was next in line, and I brought up the rear.

The horses trotted slowly, but I was too nervous to look at anything but the horse and the trail in front of me. Eventually, the first four riders pulled away from Todd and me, but we were laughing as we plodded along the trail. The leaves were deep green, and sunlight pushed through to the forest floor in shafts. We had been on the horses for maybe five minutes when I noticed that the saddle strap that hugged the belly of Todd's horse was loose. It was still laced together, but the buckle had come undone. I should have said something, but I didn't know what to say and thought maybe we would be back to the stables soon. But then the entire strap came undone.

We were in a small clearing on the trail when Todd's entire saddle flipped over onto the side of the horse. I couldn't believe what I was seeing and started screaming "Help!" Todd pulled his right foot out of the stirrup quickly, but he couldn't get his prosthetic foot free. Our horses weren't going fast, but they were going, moving forward on the trail, and I watched as Todd was dragged slowly along the forest floor. He was wearing jeans, and it looked like his left leg just kept getting longer and longer. I kept screaming for help but kept my horse behind Todd's. That's when it happened: Todd's prosthetic leg popped out of his jeans. The horse took a couple steps forward but then stopped. I stopped my horse and stared at Todd, convinced that he was dead. It seemed like time stopped. I screamed and screamed, although what I have no idea. Then Todd sat up, looked at his prosthetic leg, which was still dangling from the stirrup, and started laughing.

It was the laugh of a maniac. It was full and loud and true. He kept laughing while I yelled for everyone to come back, to help. He was still laughing by the time they had circled back, and slowly, we all started laughing hysterically. It was like Todd had just experienced the greatest thing in his life, like death had taken another shot and failed yet again, and he loved every minute of it.

That night we helped set up the community room for the dance and pizza party. We helped the DJ, who certainly had an aroma about him that someone said smelled like pot, set up his equipment. Then we took all of the pizza that had been delivered to camp and started handing it out to campers as they came into what was now a dance hall. Once the dance was cranking, we swiped two boxes of pizza and took them to the pottery workshop that was just off the main hall where the dance was taking place. We sat on the floor and someone pulled out a deck of cards. There were six of us, although Todd was not there. He was busy regaling everyone in the dance about his epic horse ride from earlier in the day. Instead, we were joined by Jason, a fifteen-year-old camper who had survived his cancer several years ago and looked completely healthy.

Someone had said we should play euchre, so we divided up into three teams. I was paired with Melissa. Ben played with Sharon, and Jason and Kim teamed up. We sat and played cards, ate pizza, and talked for what seemed like most of the night. I don't remember how Melissa and I fared as a team when it came to euchre. I knew the game pretty well. My parents and their friends would have long euchre games every weekend, and we had started playing the game at school in downtime. I don't know if Melissa was any good or not. It didn't matter, though, who won. We all spent that time together in that small space, away from all the racket of the camp itself, just a group of teenagers doing things any other groups of teenagers would have done given the circumstances.

Melissa and I talked more about being sick, about trying to recover. We were the only two in the group who were still receiving treatments, and so we talked about Dr. Koufos, the man who was directing our treatment and recovery. We talked about how nice he was, how smart. We talked about the nurses and probably said something about Ben's mom, Pam, who also was at camp that weekend and who was one of the best nurses in clinic.

Melissa talked about how excited she was to be going to the Zanesville branch of Ohio University in the fall for her first year of college. She was going to be taking foreign language and business classes, and intended to get a degree in international business. She was going to move to Boston one day, to be close to her best friend.

I would be starting what should have been my junior year in high school, trying to catch up with my class so I could graduate with them. I talked about what the previous school year had been like, how it had been so easy for the first half of the year, the half that I was repeating. I knew everything that would come up in biology, English and algebra. It was incredibly easy, and I got straight As. But then the second half started, the half I had missed, and I found myself struggling to keep up. I hated the fact that all of my friends were in classes a year ahead of me, and I was stuck in classes with kids who were in my brother John's grade. But I had pushed through, had made the baseball team, and had tried to hang out with my friends as if nothing had changed.

Going into the fall of 1992, I knew I was going to finish high school in three years and graduate with my class. My plan was to double up on the subjects that needed four classes to graduate, which was mainly math. That fall, I would be in sophomore English, sophomore geometry, and algebra II, a junior-level class, with my friends.

I would go from being a sophomore to a senior the next time we all got together at Camp CHOPS, I said. We were all sure that if the hot-air balloon we had stood in the night before was our life, it was going to soar off into the sky. We were all going to do great things, and we were itching to do them.

We made plans to get together again after camp. Melissa drove up to Apple Creek from Millersburg and picked me up in a big white car that she named Mel. The car was glistening white with light effects underneath. She had gotten it through Wishes Can Happen, an organization that grants wishes to really sick kids. I had also gotten a car from Wishes Can Happen, but had chosen an entirely economical 1987 Ford Escort, sport edition. From my house, we drove about twenty-five minutes to Marshallville to pick up Jason. Then we drove up to Cleveland to Kim's house, where Ben and Sharon were already hanging out.

We went to Dairy Queen and got ice cream, and then went back to Kim's house, where we played pinball in her basement, and then all settled on a couch to watch a movie. I sat next to Melissa, and willed myself to just brush up against her. In the end, it was only our legs that touched, but that was all right for me. What I saw in Melissa was someone who had lived almost the same experience that I had, who understood what it meant, as a teenager, to have a life-and-death struggle, to fight a disease you never could have expected would fall upon a kid. Before I got sick, I was just starting to think of myself as something more than just a fragile child. I was starting to feel indestructible as most teens do, until I was destroyed. I went from thinking nothing could stop me from becoming the future second baseman of the Chicago Cubs to wondering if life was even worth continuing. I went from wanting a girlfriend more than anything to wanting to just go home and sleep in my own bed. I went from worrying about whether the clothes I wore to school would make me look cool to wondering if I would ever go back to school.

Melissa knew all of this too. We had exchanged phone numbers at camp and occasionally talked on the phone. Melissa was the type of person who would talk to anyone on the phone for hours at a time. She frequently spent the evenings on the phone, helping friends and sometimes nonfriends with their homework, talking them through the math problems they couldn't figure out or science definitions. I wasn't used to talking on the phone a whole lot, but I had gotten some practice with my first real girlfriend, a girl I dumped just before we started our freshman year together for reasons I am still not sure of. I was most often the one who called Melissa. I usually got a busy signal, but when it went through, we would talk for a while, rehashing the types of things we had experienced and wondering what we were supposed to do with the knowledge that came from those experiences.

Melissa knew what it was like to have strangers stare at her because she had no hair and because her glasses, which looked perfectly normal on her face six months ago, now made her look like a frog because her face had sunken in so much and her eyes had become less eye-like. She knew what it was like to walk on a sidewalk and pick her knees up as high as she could, to walk like a stork, no matter how odd it made her look. She knew what it was like to fall in front of a group of people. She knew what it was like to pull clumps of hair out of her head, to wake up to thousands of strands of hair clinging to her pillow in the morning. She knew what it was like to vomit and feel the relief, if only for a few precious seconds. She knew, at the age of seventeen, what it was like to question God, to be angry at him. She knew all this, and she had processed it just like I had. We lived as teenagers who no longer believed in invincibility, but who also at times felt that we had beaten death.

She knew this, and I loved her for it.

CHAPTER 12

Good Morning America

Tim was walking outside in the bright, hot sun outside of Akron Children's one day in late July or early August of 1992 and talking with a man dressed in a suit. I stood off to the side and watched as the two talked about *Road to Remission*. Several of us, Todd included, had been called up to the hospital to participate in a news video on the game. The hospital hoped this video, which would be distributed as a news segment to TV stations around the country, would promote the board game that Tim had created and seven of us had contributed to.

I showed up at the hospital and spent a lot of time standing around and waiting until I was needed. The reporter did interviews, both inside and outside, with Tim and Kathy Parks, a child life specialist at the hospital. They walked up and down the brick sidewalk that was outside the new main entrance to the hospital. The hospital had undergone a transformation in the eighteen months since I lived there. It was newer, more vibrant.

I was also newer and more vibrant. My body had filled back out, and I weighed close to what I did when I entered the hospital. My skin was back to its normal complexion. My hair had returned, and I was growing it long. It fell out of the back of the Florida Marlins baseball cap I wore that day, the curls a bit tighter than they were before I got sick, the hair itself a bit rougher, a bit darker. But it was there, and that was all that mattered. Most importantly, I felt strong.

Eventually, six of us—Tim, Todd, Sharon, myself, and two younger kids—went into a conference room inside the hospital and started playing the game.

We went around and around and around. Drawing cards and reading them and then offering some sort of commentary on the card.

"Your parents bring you your favorite food. Go forward two spaces," Tim said at one point.

"Yaaaay!" one of the younger kids said in an incredibly soft voice.

"It would be nice if you could eat," Tim said, and we all agreed.

How many times had someone brought us food that we desperately wanted, only to take one bite and realize that the drugs had done something to our taste buds, and what was once our favorite food now tasted like cardboard or metal or worse.

We laughed a lot because the cards themselves could be funny, at least to us, because we made jokes about everything we had experienced. We had to make light of the situation because otherwise it was just too dark.

At one point, Todd drew a card and flapped his lips.

"Sick all day," he said. "Go back three spaces."

And then he laughed and we all laughed.

I drew a card that said "CT scan set back. Go back one space," and I thought about all of the CT scans I had and the infection on my brain.

After about an hour of playing the game, we were told we could stop. The news crew had gotten all the video they needed. The game was packed up and we all went home.

A few months later, a videocassette showed up in the mail. It was labeled "Today's Breakthroughs #543 Cancer Game." I popped it in the VCR that we had hooked up to the television in our basement and watched the ninety-second segment. Later, when Mom and then Dad got home, we all watched it, laughed, and talked about how I was famous now that I was on television. I watched it and was obsessed with how much I showed up on the screen. There was one shot where my arm reaches in and draws a card and then shows it to the camera. I knew it was my arm because of the mole on my right hand. That was the card that mentioned a CT scan setback. There's another shot where the camera lingers on me, a tight shot of just my face, and in the three seconds that I'm taking up the entire screen, I break into a big smile, the result, no doubt, of something Todd said.

The reporter ended the segment with this voiceover.

"Tim often worries that his cancer will come back, even though it's now in remission. His friends are not so lucky. Some have already died. Others no doubt will. He hopes his own road to remission is a journey he makes only once."

I answered the phone at our house in Apple Creek. It was a Monday or a Tuesday, the last week in October, and I had just gotten home from school. It had been three months since we made the video segment on *Road to Remission,* and even less time since the videocassette had arrived in the mail. On the other end of the line was Nancy, my social worker from the hospital. She said she had bad news.

"Todd Seitz passed away on Sunday," Nancy said.

What did I say in response? I don't know. Probably "Oh." No one had ever called me or even sat me down and told me someone had died. I didn't know what to say. Ultimately, I thanked Nancy for calling and giving me the news. I hung up, placed the phone on its base, and just sat on the stairs, lost in thoughts I never imagined I would think. The last time I had seen Todd had been when we taped the segment for *Road to Remission.* He seemed perfectly fine then. He was his normal, laughing self. I thought of Camp CHOPS, just five months earlier, when he fell off the horse. Before he fell off the horse, or maybe it was after, Todd and I had gone to the parking lot at camp to show each other our cars. He had a Ford Ranger pickup truck that he got from Wishes Can Happen. I had the Ford Escort with a sunroof and a spoiler. We joked about how easy it was to get a free car. All we had to do was get cancer.

It was hard to believe he was gone. I didn't know what I was supposed to do with that knowledge.

According to an *Akron Beacon Journal* story that was written about Todd, he had spent his last day sitting in a recliner and playing video games, yelling and carrying on with friends.

"Around suppertime, he said he was too full to eat and started coughing," the story, written by Regina Brett, says. "A few hours later, he died."

He died three weeks after his seventeenth birthday and less than five months after falling off a horse at Camp CHOPS. Two days before he died, the pastor of Todd's family's church visited.

"Are you ready for heaven?" the pastor asked Todd.

"I can never say I will ever be ready," Todd answered. "I have hope, and without hope, you have nothing."

"It was a peaceful death," his mother, Joan, told Brett. "Even to the end, he did not want to give up. He loved life."

On the morning of March 3, 1993, I stayed home from school. I was in the basement setting up the VCR to start recording channel 23 at 8 a.m. I grabbed a cassette from the wooden shelves that lined our basement wall, a cassette that I had recorded episodes of *The Simpsons* over something my brother Jim had originally recorded, and shoved it in the VCR.

Sometime in the eight o'clock hour, *Good Morning America* would have a segment on *Road to Remission*. Somehow, producers there had seen the news segment we recorded almost a year earlier, and they wanted Joan Lunden to interview Tim and someone from Akron Children's Hospital. At about 8:06 a.m., after Mark Johnson had done the local Akron weather, the station kicked it back to GMA. Lunden started the segment off by describing how a group of patients came up with a novel way to help kids with cancer, and then the camera pulled back and there was Tim, sitting in New York City on national television, alongside Lunden and Cheryl Linrode, one of the social workers at the hospital.

I sat close to the TV and stared at the screen. Tim was wearing a black-and-white-checked sweater over a dress shirt. His head was shaved, which is what prompted Lunden's first question. She wanted to know if he was all right, or if his bald head meant that he was sick with cancer again.

"I'm in great physical shape now," Tim said.

"So this was done on purpose, for the swim team, not because of chemotherapy?" Lunden asks.

"No," Tim says. "It has nothing to do with that."

"So you're feeling good?"

"I'm feeling great."

I was also feeling great. My central line had already been pulled out, and in just about two weeks, I would be done with chemotherapy and all other treatments. I was technically a sophomore in high school, but had gotten back into a lot of the junior classes with my friends and was on pace to graduate with my class. I was on the varsity baseball team, and while I wasn't a starter, I was getting to play more than I had the previous year. There were also times when I did go down to the JV team and start. In one game, I had two hits, including a double, and scored a run. I was making catches in the outfield. My hair was long enough again to hang out of my hats. One could look at me and never know, from just appearances, that I had ever been sick. That's also how Tim looked on national television.

Lunden asked about the game's creation, and Tim told the story of how when he went into the hospital after being told he had cancer, there was nothing he could relate to. He didn't understand what was happening to him, and he wondered if there was a way to make a cancer diagnosis more understandable for a kid. Lunden asked Cheryl how the game could help patients and their families. Eventually, Lunden pulls a card and reads it. As she does, I start praying that the card she is about to read is one that I wrote. I want more than anything to go to school later that day and brag about the fact that something I had written was read on national television.

"All right," Lunden said. "For instance, this is a positive card. The doctor takes the time to really listen. That must be an important one."

Not mine, I think, although it very well could have been, had I written it with the perspective I had now, the knowledge of just how special Dr. Alex Koufos was, the way he looked at me, answered all my questions, made me feel like I was not only the most important person in the room, but the most important person on the planet.

And then another: "You make a great bald joke," Lunden says. Maybe mine, I think, although when I was writing the cards, I was not of the mindset where I could find being bald funny. There was one time, though, long after we had made the game, when I sat in biology class, and the teacher, Mr. McMullen, was about to give us a quiz. He always had two versions of his quizzes, and he would let someone in the class choose quiz A or quiz B. This was in the fall of 1991, when I had returned to school for the first time. I was bald and wore a hat all day long. On this day, Mr. McMullen said, "Whoever has the best hair in the class gets to pick the quiz."

I shot my hand up immediately.

"I have the best hair. Period."

Everyone laughed. Great bald joke. I picked the quiz.

After Lunden read the bald card, everyone at the table laughed.

"Do you guys practice them?" Lunden said. "Because otherwise, you go back out to the regular school and you encounter people."

"Well, there's a whole bunch of people that don't understand it," Tim said, "and so naturally they stare, and if you just make fun of it, it's just an easy way to look at it. We, none of us were really embarrassed about our heads. We all took it in stride."

Then Lunden read some of the bad cards. Here, I thought, was my chance, considering most of the cards I wrote were negative.

"Here's a bad one, er, uh, a negative one," Lunden says. "Nurse wakes you up in the middle of the night to take your temperature."

Finally! I tried to add "and smells like cigarette smoke," when I wrote that card, but they couldn't let that stay in the game. I was so excited. I felt like a celebrity, even though my name was not on the card. Still, I would make sure everyone at school knew that I wrote that exact card.

"That's a very common one if you ask any kid in the hospital," said Tim, who was handling the interview like a professional, like he had been doing this type of thing his entire life, and not like a scared sixteen-year-old. "They're in every hour to take your blood pressure and stuff, and it always seems like it's right when you get to bed."

"Here's another," Lunden said as she pulled a card. "Another patient you know dies. That's gotta be really tough, too."

"Yeah, that's really unfortunate," Tim said, "because five of the kids that designed this game also have died since the time we designed it."

They talked a bit more about some of the good cards. Lunden read one about talking your doctor into postponing treatment so you could go to prom. I thought, as I watched, *that was Laura Jo's card.* She had talked about that in one of our support group meetings, and as I thought that, I started missing the support group. We hadn't met in a while, mainly because of what Tim had just said a few seconds ago, the part about other patients dying.

"Well," Lunden said as she started to end the segment, "now it's a real game. And we also want to point out that we have photos of the other children who contributed to this game. They include Michael Gray and Matthew Tullis, who I should say are currently doing well. All right, and also, we have five of the children who have since died, whose parents are watching this morning, and we'd like to give a special tribute to Todd Seitz, Terri Morris, Laura Jo Mounsey, John Lamb, and Shelby Lieb. You leave a contribution that will help others."

I looked at the faces of my friends, and my excitement over seeing my own face on TV drained. It left me. I went from total elation to desolation in the span of just a couple seconds. Of course, I knew they had all died, but I hadn't expected to see their faces so quickly after seeing my own, hadn't expected that immediate juxtaposition of life versus death. We were all on 4-North at the same time. We had the same nurses. We were kids thrown into a chaotic universe when we should have been spending nights at friends' houses, making prank calls, toilet-papering teachers' houses, when we should have been participating on sports teams and worrying about our grades and maybe, just maybe, starting to think about college. And not all of us got to do that. Sure, I would still go to school in a few minutes and brag about having been on national television. Sure, I would brag about having something I had written read by Joan Lunden. I would bathe in the celebrity this would give me at my tiny, rural high school. But it wouldn't be quite as glorious as

I had initially thought it would. I had spent the last two years trying to be a normal teenager again, and now I was starting to wonder if that was possible, because a normal teen wouldn't know that many people who had died at such a young age.

CHAPTER 13

Road to Remission, Interrupted

On Friday, August 27, 1994, Mom and Dad followed me to Ashland University in our brown minivan, the one that had made so many trips to Akron Children's over the last three years. The minivan was packed with several boxes of my stuff, along with a word processor and a refrigerator that would go in my dorm room. I had graduated the previous June with my class and spent the summer working in a factory to make some money to help pay for the private liberal arts education I was about to receive.

After we had carried everything up to the third floor of Kem Hall, the only male floor in a six-floor, coed building, we had lunch. Then I said good-bye to them. As Dad backed the van out of its parking spot, Mom rolled her window down. She was near tears.

"I love you," she said, and I knew she meant it. She had spent so much time and energy making sure I survived. They pulled away and I was on my own.

That night, I drank my first beer. And my second. I did a lot of orientation stuff on Saturday and Sunday and hung out with some people from my high school who had also gone to AU. There were four of us from Waynedale, but I was the only guy. I knew I wouldn't see those young women much once classes started because I had decided to major in journalism and they had not. That was fine with me because I really preferred that people at Ashland not know about what now seemed like a past life.

I was better. I was alive. I was starting a new life. I was getting stronger, and because of that, I failed to see that others, those I cared a great deal about, were weakening.

Monday, August 30, was my first day of classes at Ashland University. The day included a Western civilization class with an old Italian professor who cussed a lot (and who, rumor had it, had jumped out of a second-floor classroom window the previous year because the students weren't listening to him), and an intro to political thought class taught by a man who worked in Ronald Reagan's White House.

While I was taking all that in, and trying to forget the last three years of my life, my nurse Janet died in her Orrville home. She had been battling cancer for nearly two years. I had been told on a clinic visit that Janet had cancer when she was initially diagnosed, back in 1992. But I hadn't seen her since the last time she was my nurse, which would have been sometime that summer of 1991, when I was in the hospital for an extended chemotherapy drip.

For Janet, it started in October 1992, when she called her husband Dennis from Akron Children's and told him she was unable to go to the bathroom. They thought it might be irritable bowel syndrome, but a visit to the doctor ultimately revealed a massive tumor on her gall bladder. She was told she had adenocarcinoma. She needed to see an oncologist, and she got in to Memorial Sloan Kettering Cancer Center, one of the best places in the world to go for cancer treatment. Even then, she was told she had just a 5 percent chance at being cured. She lived for twenty-two months.

During those twenty-two months, she continued working at the hospital. She lost her hair because of the chemotherapy, just like so many of her patients had, and instead of wearing a wig, she wore a bandana.

I don't remember exactly how I learned that Janet died, although the most likely way was that Mom called me in my dorm room when she saw the obituary in the local newspaper. I thought, how could a woman who took care of kids with cancer ultimately die of cancer? In what world was this even a possibility?

I spent that first semester trying to be a completely normal college student. I went to parties on the weekend. I got incredibly drunk for the first time and, simultaneously, threatened to beat up a varsity baseball player, a young man who was six-feet, two-inches tall and weighed about a hundred pounds more than me. I started immediately working for the student newspaper and found myself covering the university's football games. I went to the games and then showed up every Monday morning to interview the head coach. I wrote stories about soccer as well, even though I had never been to a soccer match before.

I went to my classes, or most of them, but had a hard time taking anything seriously. I enjoyed my exploring the Bible class, primarily because it opened my eyes into how the book was put together. Western civilization was amazing because nobody ever knew what was going to come out of Charles Ferroni's mouth. But Spanish? That political thought class? I struggled through them, got low Cs, but I didn't really care.

The class I rarely went to was English 101. The class was held every Tuesday and Thursday at 8 a.m., and the professor didn't take attendance. I turned in the first paper, a five-page essay on Ray Bradbury's "The Veldt," focused on why Bradbury has the children in the story using the word "coldly" in describing how they talk to their parents. I wrote it the night before it was due. I thought it was awesome. Dr. Weaver gave it back to me a week later with an F in the top left, and the words "too journalistic" written on the back. I stopped going to class after that, and ultimately failed the class.

After the second worst semester of my life (the first being the one I spent in the hospital), one that left me with a sterling 1.9 GPA, I went home for Christmas break. There was a stack of *Daily Record* newspapers waiting for me in my bedroom when I got there. I had asked Mom and Dad to save the papers for me so I could read them whenever I came home. I was majoring in journalism, was going to be a newspaper reporter one day, and while I blew off a lot of my classes, I wanted to devour all the news that I could.

I turned on the television in my bedroom and sat down on the blue carpet. I picked up the newspapers, one by one, and started reading them the way I always did, by scanning the obituary listings. I had started doing this a few years earlier, after I got out of the hospital and knew that death was real. I always wanted to know how old the people who had died that week were, whether they had been able to live a long life, or whether theirs was cut short, like mine almost had been. Then I flipped through the paper, stopping to read whatever sounded interesting. I don't know how many papers I had read before one stuck a knife in my heart. I picked it up and looked at the obituary listings on the front page.

Melissa Lanning, 21.

In June 1993, our CIT group at Camp CHOPS was back, mostly. We were missing Todd, but everyone else was there. Melissa, Ben, Sharon, Kim, and me. I went to that camp just about three months after my final clinic visit as a patient who was receiving chemotherapy. I was seventeen years old and weighed 125 pounds, finally back to where I was when I got sick more than two years earlier. My blood pressure was strong, at 116 over 68.

"Doing well," Dr. Koufos wrote in his physician's notes. "Appetite, activity good."

During this visit, Dr. Koufos performed one final spinal tap, injecting two milligrams of vincristine into my spine. At home after that visit, I took prednisone and methotrexate orally for one week. I took my final pill on March 14 and was officially "off therapy."

The central line was also gone from my chest. A few months earlier, Dr. Andrews, the man who had inserted it, came into an exam room in a different part of the hospital after I had already visited the clinic. He pulled and pulled and pulled and then it just popped out. No more dressing changes. I could now take showers, and I took one when I got home from clinic that day, my first shower since the morning of January 2, 1991. I scrubbed at all the accumulated dirt and adhesive that had built up around the central line's dressing. The hot water—I had turned it up as hot as it would go—poured over me, and I scrubbed like I had never scrubbed before, trying to wash away as much of the past two years as possible.

Melissa was finishing up her first year as a college student when she came back to Camp CHOPS that year, and she said she loved it. She was taking the types of classes she told us she was going to take the previous summer. She had gotten great grades in the fall and winter quarters and expected the same this time around. There was no way any of us could have known as we spent that weekend together that the cancer was already growing in Melissa's body, that she would never take her final exams and never finish college.

She came back to camp again in 1994, so at some point that weekend, if not on a phone call before, I found out she had relapsed. But what did we talk about at camp that weekend? Did we talk about her relapse? Did she tell us she was going to die? I have no memories of any such discussions, only one of being completely shocked when I saw her obituary, like her death was one I never thought would happen.

I kept her phone number on my bulletin board but never called even though I knew she was sick. Was I afraid of talking to someone who knew her time on this planet was going to end soon? Or was I frightened by the fact that we could get better and then unbetter, and talking to Melissa would have forced that knowledge to the front of my brain? Or maybe I was just having too much fun trying to be a normal college kid, and talking to her would make me acknowledge that I wasn't normal, that I never would be.

I sat there, staring at the newspaper, blinking back tears. I tried to read the words on her obituary, tried to make sense of what had happened. I had always viewed Melissa as somewhat of my clone, the person who was more like me than any other person on the planet. We were close to the same age.

We grew up in small towns not far from each other. We both had childhood cancer, and we both had Dr. Alex Koufos working to save us. I started wondering why she wasn't sitting in her bedroom reading my obit.

I stood up and walked to my car. I felt robotic. I knew I had to do something, and I desperately wanted to feel something, but I could access nothing but complete and utter numbness. I drove less than a mile to the Apple Creek Town & Country store, which at the time was the only place to buy greeting cards in the village. I picked out what was probably the only sympathy card available, bought it, and then drove home. There, I opened the card and wrote something inside, something generic like, "Sorry for your loss." I sealed it up and put Melissa's mom's name and address on it. I put a stamp in the corner and walked it out to the mailbox.

There would be times later in my life when I would think about writing in that card and wish I could have a do over. Sometimes, I wish I would have written, "I'm sorry it wasn't me," or "I wish I had called," or "This is fucking bullshit." But mostly I think about the first alternate possibility. What would Melissa have done in life had she not relapsed? Would she have done more for this world than I have? How can I justify my survival? How can I live so I'm not sorry it wasn't me?

I didn't go to the calling hours or her funeral, although now, twenty-four years later, I don't know why. Perhaps I just couldn't take it. It was too close to home. I hadn't gone to Todd's funeral either. Melissa's death shook me in a way Todd's hadn't, and I had no idea how to grapple with the state it left me in. And so I pushed it down, I buried the thoughts that came into my brain. I put the card in the mail and tried to go on living my life like I was perfectly normal.

CHAPTER 14

Orrville

I n the summer of 1995, I worked second shift in a factory in Orrville. Every day, I drove past the street Janet used to lived on. Oftentimes, I found myself eating dinner at the McDonald's where she picked up sausage biscuits for me. That summer was a rough one. It was the summer between my freshman and sophomore years of college. I had rebounded some in the spring semester thanks to some journalism courses and no Spanish. Mom and Dad divorced in January, and so when I came home for summer break, it was the first time I had lived at home with only one parent. Additionally, my dad's new wife worked in the office of the factory where I was working, which is mostly how I got the job. It's also the employer that my dad had driven his semi for throughout my childhood, the exact building where we spent our Saturdays as kids, riding our bikes and having a picnic lunch while Dad worked on his truck.

I spent most of that summer drunk and in a haze. It's easy enough to pin the blame on my parents' divorce, but that's lazy. There was more to it than that. I was, of course, about to be a sophomore in college. In high school, a time when so many kids get their first tastes of beer, I had just one sip, at a restaurant with my friend's family. Doctors were too busy pouring other things that completely changed the way I felt into my body at the time, so alcohol didn't seem all that appealing.

But by the time I got to college, things changed. I had changed but wasn't yet willing to acknowledge it. I lived the life of a college student, as if I were no different from anyone else. I went to off-campus parties. I drank Zima and warm Miller Lite and Red Dog and whatever beer anyone put in front of me. By the time my parents split, I was driving home on the weekends to hang out with high school friends and get shitfaced on bottles of Mad Dog 20/20 and cases of Pabst Blue Ribbon beer.

By the time the summer rolled around, my liver was marinating in chemicals in a way it hadn't since my first days in the hospital. I worked second shift, often from 3 p.m. until 11 p.m., pulling big boxes of cardboard tubes off a conveyer belt and stacking them on pallets. It was a hot summer, and the job was grueling. Often, I worked a twelve-hour shift, and even more often, after work, I would head out to a bar with some of the older workers and drink a beer or two before heading home. On the weekends, my high school friends and I would drive to Canton, to a shopping mall that was no more than a couple miles from Dr. Koufos's house (although I didn't know this at the time), and we would each chug six bottles of Bud Ice (highest alcohol content we could find) and then walk blitzed into a dance club, knowing our drunkenness wouldn't subside until last call and it was time to head home.

On the outside, at least to people who knew me, it probably looked like I was trying to finish the job that cancer had started. Internally, I don't know what I was trying to accomplish. My days were spent going to work in a place that was a memorial to my parents' divorce. One tow motor operator came up to me once and told me about how devastated my dad looked before the divorce, when he came into the factory. She said he just didn't know what to do. And then she told me he was so much happier now. My inclination was to tell the woman to fuck off and that I didn't care what she or anyone thought, much as I had told Mom and Dad when they told me they were getting a divorce. So maybe the drinking was partly because of where I spent my days. But I think it also had to do with the town of Orrville itself.

I couldn't drive to work that summer without thinking about being sick. When I went to the hospital, it was through Orrville. I had been driving through that town and past the factory where I now worked hundreds of times on my way to spinal taps, hospital stays and terrible, four-hour chemotherapy drips that left me feeling like I had been run over by the semi my dad drove on a daily basis. There was the McDonald's that Mom and I would stop at on our way home from hospital visits, the one that Janet stopped at on her way to work. I thought about Janet constantly, and that made me think about Melissa and Todd. How could a nineteen-year-old who was pretending that nothing had ever happened to him handle all of those memories, all of those ghosts?

One day, it was unbearably hot and humid. I had to wear jeans and steel-toed boots to work, and at this time, my hair was long enough to be pulled back into a ponytail, which made everything feel even hotter. On this day, though, a severe storm moved through. It knocked out power and we were told on the factory floor that there was a tornado warning. We started hearing pings, like something hitting the metal walls of the factory. I walked over to a door that opened up to the back of the building and pushed through it. It was an incredibly stupid thing to do, but I've always been drawn to severe storms. It had been so dry that summer, and dirt was swirling all around. I could see lightening and hear loud cracks of thunder. The pinging, I realized, was hail. The sky was about to be ripped open, and while we wouldn't get a tornado, we did get the type of Ohio thunderstorm that makes you wonder if you'll survive. I found that I was craving that feeling, that uncertainty.

I somehow survived both that storm and the year of drunken bitterness. I don't know exactly how or why it stopped, other than the fact I met a girl (a girl who would one day become my wife) who pulled all the warm, unstable air out of me, causing my desire to hide who I was to dissipate. Now that I finally stopped pretending that nothing bad had happened to me, I started writing about it.

CHAPTER 15

Final Visit

I crossed the bridge from the parking garage into Akron Children's Hospital the morning of December 19, 1997. I carried a blue composition notebook in my hand and a determination in my mind to know just how sick I had been. I had just finished the fall semester of my senior year at Ashland University. I started taking college a bit more seriously after that summer in Orrville, and my grades improved dramatically. I was the co-editor-in-chief of the student newspaper and often found myself writing about my illness in philosophy classes, advanced composition classes, and creative writing classes. I was one semester away from graduating from college and envisioned writing a book about being sick.

It had been nearly seven years since I entered Akron Children's Hospital as a kid who was only a couple weeks away from dying because my blood had gone bad. I needed a checkup with Dr. Koufos, but I also thought it would be nice to talk to him about my sickness. When I asked if he would spend some time talking to me, he, of course, said yes, because he always said yes to questions like that.

The clinic was different now. It was no longer located in that dank hallway on the second floor. Now it was on the fifth floor, with windows that looked out upon downtown Akron. The waiting room was bursting with color, blues and purples and greens everywhere, on the walls, on the carpet. There was a huge fish tank and a tiny room that looked like a tree house that only little kids could squeeze into. There was a television. There were books and games and comfortable chairs. And while the clinic was always just called the clinic when I was a regular patient, this space also had an official name now, the Showers Family Center for Childhood Cancer and Blood Disorders.

Dr. Koufos wrote in my chart, "22 year old white male diagnosed 1/91 T-Cell ALL." "Prescribed Regimen B 1901. To finish college this year. Doing well. Remains alert, active. No complaints."

I weighed 170 pounds when I stepped on the scale. I was shaving my head now, but only because that was a look I wanted. I realized after having the ponytail for about a year that the look wasn't my best. I also no longer felt the need to have long hair to make me forget about the days when I had no hair.

Dr. Koufos was also different. He was thinner, much thinner than I had ever seen him. He didn't look sick, at least not to me, but I knew he was. He had been fighting a rare form of cancer in his bile duct for more than a year.

"How's Mom and Dad?" he asked.

"They're good," I said.

"Your brothers?

"Also good."

"How are you feeling?"

I told Dr. Koufos that I was feeling great. I had a girlfriend. I was doing well in college. I had, as so many nurses had written in my charts on my good days in the hospital, "no complaints."

Dr. Koufos put the stethoscope in his ears.

"This is cold," he said. "Sorry."

Then he placed it against my back and listened to my lungs. They were clear. Then he put it on my chest.

"Your heart is strong," he said. "That's good."

After my checkup, Dr. Koufos and I sat down at a table in a room that was remarkably similar to the one in which my parents and I met with him nearly seven years earlier, when he laid out the treatment that would save my life. That was the meeting in which Dr. Koufos told my parents and me exactly what my body was in for, the meeting in which he told us I had a very poor prognosis, that I very well might die.

I didn't, though, because of this man. Today, he was quieter than usual, although he was never loud in the first place. His eyes were softer too, although they were never hard.

He looked at me and said, "It's different, isn't it? It really changes you."

I knew that he was talking about cancer.

For so long, Dr. Koufos had been as much of a god to me as the one I believed in as a kid at church. He was the man who saved my life, who not only saved me but breathed new life into me when there was nothing left but a bunch of mutant white blood cells running around my body. But now, we were equals. He looked at me in a way I hadn't seen before, like he had finally figured out what all of us childhood cancer patients already knew but hadn't recognized yet, and this knowledge gave him a better understanding of everything he had done in life. In that moment, when he looked at me and saw not a fifteen-year-old boy whose eyes were sunken into his head or a boy who wanted to lie in bed until he permanently went to sleep, but instead saw a healthy twenty-two-year-old man who was ready to live, who was living, he must have understood the miracles he performed, and that changed him too. And he must have realized there was no miracle coming for him.

At the time, I was obsessed with a confirmation that I was a special person, that I had survived something I shouldn't have. I wanted a dramatic story arc to my first writings about having survived cancer because I thought that was what would sell, that was what would make me the famous author I had always wanted to be. So many people had told me I was special over the last six years, that I was a miracle and proof of God's work in our lives, and now I needed that medical confirmation from the man who saved my life.

Dr. Koufos had the six volumes of medical records I had accumulated in front of him, and he flipped through them. The first volume had a bunch pages with numbers upon numbers upon numbers that only made sense to a doctor or a nurse. The second volume, which he was flipping through now, had nursing flow charts and his physician's notes. Was he reminiscing? Was he looking for answers to the question of how I survived? Was there anything in there that could tell him why others didn't? He didn't say much.

"We threw a lot at you," he said.

He only had five more months to live, although he and I didn't know that. I thought about his words: it changes you. Eventually, a wave of clarity would wash over me, and I would come to realize it didn't matter how sick I was. The only thing that mattered was that I was alive. As a teenager, a high schooler, and then a college student, I had worked so hard to get back to "normal" while simultaneously trying to convince people that I was special. I had worked so hard to graduate with my own high school class, to fit in with my friends, to go to college and pretend that nothing had ever happened to me, that I failed to realize that I was different, that I had changed. The Matt Tullis who entered Akron Children's Hospital on January 4, 1991, was dead, only I didn't realize this until much later. A new Matt Tullis had taken his place, one who, if he thought about it for one second, knew he experienced life in a different way.

"How sick was I?"

I was still fixated on something that was meaningless.

Dr. Koufos chuckled.

"You were one sick cookie."

The man who saved my life became jaundiced and fatigued in November 1996. He went in for tests, thinking he had hepatitis or something similar. Doctors at Akron General did a biopsy of his liver. Just a few days before Thanksgiving, the diagnosis came back. Cholangiocarcinoma. It's a cancer of the bile ducts, which drain bile from the liver into the small intestine. It is rare, with only one to two cases per one hundred thousand people being reported in North America. It is considered incurable, with the median survival rates (for the type of cancer Dr. Koufos had) being six months. Of course, as an oncologist, he knew all of this the second he saw the diagnosis. He knew he had been sentenced to an early death.

He kept pushing, though, living longer than expected and continuing to see patients from time to time, including me in December 1997.

In March 1998, Alex developed an infection. He went to Akron General Hospital feeling sick. X-rays showed the cancer hadn't spread anywhere else, and talk of a transplant was revived. He was airlifted to Pittsburgh where he was put on the transplant list. The infection and the medication to fight the infection took its toll. Before the treatment, doctors told Dr. Koufos and his wife Kathy that the medication was aggressive, and it would affect his kidneys and other organs. He told his wife that without the medication, the infection would kill him.

"This at least gives me a chance," he said to her.

Ultimately, as he lay in a hospital room in Pittsburgh, two-and-a-half hours east of his hometown of Canton, his kidneys shut down. His three children were by his side up until the final two hours, when a grandmother whisked them away. Then Kathy sat beside her husband until he died at 5:10 p.m. on April 26, 1998. He was 45 years old.

I was in my dorm room, getting ready for class—my nonfiction workshop—when the phone rang. It was Nancy, the social worker. She told me that Dr. Koufos had passed away, and I thanked her for calling me, for telling me. When I left the clinic after visiting with Dr. Koufos in December, he told me he wanted to see me again in one year. He had even written that down my records. I had told him I would be back before then, to go over my records more closely, and he said he would be more than happy to do that with me. But I never went back, and now he was dead.

I hung up the phone and sat down on my bed and cried. I cried like I've only cried a handful of times in my life, deep sobs followed by desperate gasps for air, all done with the effort of understanding exactly what this all meant. I cried because Dr. Koufos would never meet the woman I was going to marry, because he wouldn't attend my college graduation. I cried because he would never meet the son I would make sure carried part of his name, and because he would never see what I would become, what I would do with the life he gave me. I cried because he was dead and I was still alive and it just didn't seem right.

PART III

GHOSTS

CHAPTER 16

Scars

I shave my head every two weeks, and in the ten years since I started doing this, I've collected a great number of scars, nineteen to be exact. Now, when I stare in the mirror and sheer off the meager stubs of hair that push through my scalp, I uncover the marks. The scars are the result of basal cell carcinoma, a minor form of skin cancer that is treated by removing it surgically. The procedure is done on an outpatient basis. Every year, my dermatologist spots three or four more and sets me up with a surgeon who will make more scars.

The first one showed up in 2004. I was a graduate student at the University of North Carolina Wilmington. Sometime the year before, I noticed a spot on my head, by my left temple, that looked like a mole but constantly broke open and bled. It would scab up, then break open, then scab up, then break open. I knew I should get it checked out, but I didn't have a doctor or a dermatologist in Wilmington, so I let it go. Then, over the course of a handful of months, two things happened: First, I was working at Barnes & Noble when a man came up to my register with a couple of books. I rang them up, and as I did, he stared at me, at my head. I told him the total.

"Do you see a dermatologist?" he asked me as he handed me some cash.

I pushed a few keys on the register and then lied.

"Yes," I said. I hadn't seen a dermatologist in more than four years.

"Good," he said, and then walked away.

That alone made it one of the weirdest encounters I had while working retail. But then he was back a couple minutes later, with a magazine. This time, he handed me a credit card. Under his name was the name of a dermatology practice in Wilmington.

I wrote about that experience in a piece I had been working on for my creative writing workshop. I was picked to be the opening reader for Dinty

W. Moore, an essayist who had come to campus for a few days. I stood in front of a crowded auditorium and read my essay "Moles." After the reading, Dinty said I should go see a doctor.

That's ultimately what got me to Northeast Dermatology, where a painting of the practice's physicians hung on the wall in the waiting room. In the middle of that painting was the man from my Barnes & Noble cash register. I didn't see him that day, but another doctor scraped the scabbing, gross mole off my forehead while she talked with a nurse about *American Idol* and Fantasia Barrino. A couple days later, a nurse called and told me the spot was a basal cell. I was frightened at first. It was the first time a dermatologist took something off my skin that was cancerous. After doing a bit of research on the Internet, though, I felt safe knowing that type of cancer was easily treated.

And it was. A plastic surgeon cut it out and stitched me up, leaving a lightning bolt shaped scar on the left side of my forehead. This was at the height of Harry Potter mania, between J. K. Rowling's fifth and sixth installment. I liked to go around and tell people, after pointing at my scar, that I was the boy who lived. And I was, really. What I didn't tell them was how hard it was to understand what surviving meant and what I was supposed to do with the gift I had been given.

Alyssa and I married in 2000, and Emery, our son, was born in 2004, just about two months after that first basal cell was removed. We moved around a lot. We left Wilmington in 2005, heading back to Ohio, back to Wooster. And after eight months there, we packed up and moved south to Columbus, where our daughter Lily would be born. Because of the frequent moves, I never established myself with a regular physician or a dermatologist, so it was at least another two years before I finally saw a skin doctor again. This time, he found two basal cell carcinomas. He removed them and stitched me up and then six months later, he found a couple more. He became fascinated by the fact that I had now had five basal cells and I was only thirty-one. It wasn't until I mentioned that I had cranial radiation as a fifteen-year-old cancer patient that everything clicked in to place.

"Well," he said, "now this makes sense."

In April 1991, just about a month after I got out of Akron Children's Hospital, I spent ten different mornings at Akron General Hospital, so someone could point radiation beams at my skull. The radiation was supposed to kill any leukemic cells that may have crossed the blood-brain barrier. Initially, I was supposed to have had the radiation treatments in late February and early March, but they had to be postponed because of the infection on my brain. In fact, Dr. Koufos had made a presentation to a board of physicians regarding the need to hold off on radiation, and argue that I should still be kept in the treatment study group I was in.

Those days in April are mostly a blur. I initially met Dr. Mitchel Fromm at Akron General on April 3 for an evaluation. On that day, I vomited and couldn't catch my breath. I nearly passed out as I stood on a scale and had to sit down and put my head between my knees. That wasn't enough to stop the treatments, though, because six days later, Mom took me to Akron General Hospital, where a television in the waiting room seemed to always be playing *The Price Is Right*, and those first radiation waves were aimed at my head. I received ten treatments over thirteen days. The radiation was aimed at my entire brain and scorched my scalp and ears. By April 20, the treatments were done. The burns started healing. My body recovered from the nausea that was caused by the radiation. I regained the minimal energy I had managed to generate before the treatments, and I continued on with all of my other chemotherapy drugs as an outpatient. I was happy to be done with the radiation and thought I would never have to think about it again. I didn't know that it would never be done with me.

I'm forty-one years old now. Alyssa and I have been married for seventeen years. We have two amazing kids. I'm now at my second university, teaching journalism courses. I've accomplished a lot as a writer, and even more, I think, as a husband and father.

But sometimes, as I'm shaving my head, I'll stop and stare directly at one or two of the scars and think about those days in April and wonder how long the basal cell that once lived there had been incubating. And sometimes, I think far worse things, like what if there's a brain tumor in there somewhere, hiding in the folds of my brain, not yet causing any damage, but just waiting to wreck what has become an amazing life. How could there not be a brain tumor there? After all, doctors literally shot cancer-causing waves directly at my brain for ten days, and those rays have already caused nineteen minor skin cancers. Surely there is more to come.

I try not to dwell on those thoughts, though, because it seems like I am being ungrateful. I am an ungrateful survivor. Wouldn't Melissa have given anything to develop skin cancers twenty years later? Wouldn't Todd have gladly taken his chances on developing a brain tumor if it guaranteed him another two decades of life? When I look at the scars, I think of my friends, and I miss them and think they got a bad draw. My amazing life withers away in front of my eyes, and I feel like I'm not doing enough to justify my survival over their deaths. I do all of these mental calculations with the clear knowledge that those two things—my living and their dying—are not linked in any way. Still, I can't stop thinking about it that way.

When I see the scars, I also see all of the moles on my body because that's often what basal cells start off looking like. Moles dominate the landscape of my body. They are like stars in the galaxy, making up constellations on my arms and face and back. I recently visited my dermatologist—and I can finally say "my" dermatologist because I've been seeing her every six months for about five years—and as she looked over my body, she called out how many dysplastic nevi, or uncommon moles—I had on each body part. More than fifty on my back. More than thirty-five on my right arm. About fifty on my left arm. Fifteen on the right side of my face.

On my left arm, the letter P is formed in moles. Five years ago, you could take away the curve of the P and I had the first five planets of the solar system perfectly aligned, correct in scale. Now it seems Mercury has either moved or disappeared entirely. The moles on the curve of the P have gotten bigger, like a star about to go supernova.

Moles begin as benign skin spots, formed by nests of pigment forming cells. While sun exposure can increase the number of moles one has, family history is the main factor when it comes to determining whether or not you can play connect the dots on your forearm or upper back.

Once, when I was working at the *Columbus Dispatch*, I was interviewing Dr. Frederick Ruymann, a pediatric oncologist, for a story I was doing on the long-term effects of childhood cancer. During the interview, I told Dr. Ruymann that I was a childhood cancer survivor, knowing that the knowledge would allow Dr. Ruymann to speak more openly, would give him understanding that I knew a lot about the subject. He asked me who had treated me.

"Dr. Alex Koufos, at Akron Children's," I said.

"Ah, Alex," Dr. Ruymann said.

He had worked extensively with Dr. Koufos back when my doctor was in medical school, so we talked the man we both knew for a bit. Dr. Ruymann said that Alex was a gifted physician and researcher, and that it was a shame that he didn't have a full life to treat children with cancer.

Once we were done with the interview, we walked out of the massive building that was Nationwide Children's Hospital in Columbus. At the entrance of the hospital, Dr. Ruymann pulled out a pen and pointed to the moles on my face. He asked if I had ever been diagnosed with neurofibromatosis, to which I answered I had not. I hadn't even ever heard of it. He didn't explain the condition, only added that the number of moles on my body was a good sign that I had NFB, and that I should definitely see a dermatologist regularly.

I did some research that night, typing NFB into Google, and found that neurofibromatosis is typically diagnosed when a person has six or more light brown, raised spots on the skin. I had probably close to fifty that were light brown, and another two hundred that were varying shades of darker brown. I also found a study that was published in the *British Journal of Cancer* in 1994 that said, "There is a well-known raised risk of leukemia in children with neurofibromatosis type 1." My moles, all along, were warning signs, signs we didn't even know to look for, that nobody knew to look for, at least not at the time.

When I think of moles, I also think of the animal, burrowing through the ground and popping up occasionally, ruining a perfectly good lawn. I've come to view my childhood cancer, in many ways, as a mole that is constantly burrowing into my writing. When I was a newspaper reporter, I was always finding ways to write about people who had cancer, kids who had cancer, or my own cancer. In my more creative pursuits, cancer finds a way into just about everything I write.

In graduate school, I set out to write an essay about my parents' divorce, and by the end of that essay, there were several scenes that were directly related to my cancer. There was the scene of my dad sneaking into my bedroom in the middle of the night, turning on my television, and sitting in the white Rubbermaid chair we kept by my bedside. He did this several times, and for a long time, I figured he just missed those nights when I was in the hospital, when it was just the two of us in the room and a television throwing shadows against the wall. He would sit there, not realizing I was awake, or maybe realizing I was awake, and then he would get up and, I always assumed, go back to bed.

Then there was the scene that Mom described for me, when she was climbing the stairs in the parking garage, on her way to see me the day I was moved into the Intensive Care Unit, and she collapsed in the stairwell and cried out to God to not punish her through me. My parents, apparently, were close to getting a divorce when I got sick, and the guilt was eating her up. She saw my sickness as a punishment for her wanting something more out of life than what she currently had, and she couldn't take it anymore.

Cancer burrows in to everything, and I think it's because I have not yet come to terms with what I went through. I have not yet fully understood how the disease shaped my life, and how it is still shaping my life a quarter-century later.

I think about Janet, Dr. Koufos, Melissa, Todd, Tim, Terri, Laura Jo, Shelby, everyone I knew who didn't survive, when I see my scars. They had their own scars, of course, but not the scars that came with survival, scars that came with what the childhood cancer community calls late effects, the long-term side effects caused by the toxic drugs that were used to try to save our lives.

In 2007, I went back to Akron Children's with Mom, another trip to the clinic for a checkup. Dr. Koufos wasn't there, of course. And neither were Drs. Kastelic and Krill, both retired at the time. Dr. Talai was still there, along with a new army of doctors. One of the areas the clinic was now specializing in was late effects. My former nurse Pam, the one I have stayed in the most contact with, runs the clinic. On the day I went back, I took Mom instead of my wife, Alyssa. Why? Because I thought I was going to create some magic by putting Mom and me back into those clinic exam rooms together again. I thought I was going to experience what I would ultimately write as the perfect ending to a book about surviving childhood cancer.

Like the time I thought the ending to my cancer story was my base hit up the middle for the junior varsity baseball team, I was wrong. I envisioned being checked out and told I was perfectly healthy. I envisioned Mom and me driving back from Akron, just like we had done on March 8, 1993, after I had had my final official visit as a chemotherapy patient, as well as the day Dr. Andrews yanked at my central line until it popped out, and I felt like I was finally unthethered to the world of cancer. I envisioned a drive and some quiet reflection on the fact that it was all, finally, over, and that I could move on with my life and stop living in the past.

It was on this trip that I first learned that the radiation I had could ultimately cause some problems. That's why I brought it up with my dermatologist the next time I went. I learned I had some lung issues, possibly the start of chronic obstructive pulmonary disease, caused by some of the chemotherapy drugs. I learned my testosterone was low, and while that typically happens as men age, I was told my testosterone was low at an early age because of what the drugs and radiation had done to my pituitary gland. I learned that I was at risk for depression, something I no doubt laughed at, until I sank deep into my own depressed brain about five years later. I found out I was overweight, and when Pam asked me if I ever exercised, I laughed and said no. She asked if I ate healthy foods, and I said I ate whatever I felt like eating.

"I don't know why you even bothered coming in here if you're not going to take your health seriously," she said, and that stung.

Sure, my bones were strong. For now. But I needed to exercise, good heart and bone-pounding exercise. I needed to eat better and lose a lot of weight, about thirty pounds.

Fortunately, an echocardiogram showed us what Dr. Koufos had always told me on so many trips to the clinic, that my heart was strong. But would it always be that way? The way I was living? And even if I lived perfectly, that was no guarantee my life would extend to that of a normal, never-had-childhood-cancer adult. I learned that many childhood cancer survivors are now developing tumors throughout their bodies, especially those who received radiation. In an issue of the *New England Journal of Medicine*, a study was published that looked at the chronic health conditions in adult survivors of childhood cancer, and it found that among the 10,397 survivors, more than 62 percent had at least one chronic condition and 27.5 percent had a severe or life-threatening condition. One of the study's conclusions was that damage to organ systems caused by chemotherapy and radiation may not become clinically evident for years. The drugs that saved my life also planted a ticking time bomb in my body.

I never really asked the question, "Why did I get cancer?" It seemed like a foolish question to ask because, quite frankly, there wasn't an answer. Or if there is an answer now, it's one that would then necessitate more questions. Maybe I got cancer because maybe I have neurofibromatosis. And maybe one gene in my DNA blipped, malfunctioned, glitched, and started making cancer cells. But then, why might I have neurofibromatosis? Why could it cause my DNA to blip? I could dig down so far on this question and never get a satisfactory answer, and so I've never really asked it.

I've asked other questions like, *When did my bone marrow start producing mutant blood cells?* Was it there when the blood test was done before my hernia surgery? Did it show up one day when I was in algebra class, listening to Mrs.

Bergen scream at students for not getting their homework done? Or did it appear when I was at home, inhaling microwave popcorn and Mountain Dew while I watched game shows on the USA Network?

Once I started getting better, I asked myself, *What can I get away with because I'm the kid with leukemia?* and I pushed that as far as it would go. I talked back to teachers and cheated on tests. I did things that other kids would have been given in-school suspensions for. I don't ever remember being reprimanded once all through high school.

But the question I've asked the most, especially after that late effect clinic, after these cancers started showing up on my head, after I started thinking about how I would never be free of this cancer that struck me when I was just fifteen years old, is *Why did I survive, and why did everyone else die?*

I no longer believe my survival was ordained on high by some God floating in the sky. I felt that way for a long time, a feeling that was perpetuated by those in my church who claimed I was a miracle and that God had great things planned for me and for my life. As I got older, I became disillusioned with this line of thought. I wondered, why is God so callous, uncaring, and shortsighted? I remember thinking that the God I once loved was vindictive and uncaring. This was after someone told me I was really special, that God had plans for me. *Really,* I thought? He couldn't think of something awesome to do with Melissa? Or Dr. Koufos, who saved the lives of kids with cancer on a regular basis? That wasn't great enough? Because I long ago abandoned the feeling that I was kept on this planet by God to do something amazing—become president, write a next great American novel, who knows—I've struggled with this question. It's morphed from *Why did I survive?* to *What am I supposed to do with this survival?* I went from waiting for something great to happen to actively trying to figure how I could justify my survival.

I know I survived now because my cancer was in the blood, and Melissa's and Todd's and Tim's and Janet's and Dr. Koufos's was in their tissues, and tissue cancers are much harder to cure than blood cancers. I survived because my body reacted favorably to the cocktail of drugs that Dr. Koufos gave me. I survived because he was able to combine scientific knowledge with a bedside manner, and that all of the leukemic cells in my body were killed, and the bacteria on my brain was obliterated, and ultimately, my body recovered and didn't malfunction again. That's why I survived.

So now the question I ask is, *"What does all this mean?"*

CHAPTER 17

Searching For My Doctor

I sat courtside in the Schottenstein Center at The Ohio State University, the arena where the Buckeyes' basketball teams play their home games. A handful of OSU men's basketball players trickled onto the court to warm up before practice. Sitting across from me on a folding chair was a seven-foot-tall player, a nineteen-year-old whose last name was Koufos.

Kosta Koufos was a freshman on the Buckeyes at the time. He was a starter and a surefire first-round pick in the National Basketball Association's upcoming draft. The last time I had seen him, he was nine years old, dressed in a suit, and sitting in an overflowing auditorium at Akron Children's Hospital, listening to a bunch of strangers talk about how amazing his father was.

It was February 2008, and I was a reporter in the features department at the *Columbus Dispatch*. During the summer of 2007, I saw a clip on the sports page of the Dispatch about a high school kid named Kosta Koufos signing to play college basketball at Ohio State, and I wondered . . . could it be? I called Pam and asked if Kosta was my doctor's son.

"He is," she said.

I pitched a story to my editors about how when Kosta was nine, his father, a celebrated doctor at Akron Children's Hospital, a doctor who saved the lives of many children who had cancer, had himself died of cancer. I also told them that I was one of those children. I was worried my editors would say no, that I had too many connections to the family already, that my story could not be unbiased, but they didn't say that. They told me to do the story.

I contacted the OSU athletics department and convinced them to give me a one-on-one interview with Kosta. I would get about fifteen minutes before practice, and then he would need to hit the court.

I no longer have the digital voice recorder that I used for this interview, and, in a huge mistake, never saved the sound file. I'm left with the notes from the interview as well as the story, which ran at just under a thousand words in the *Columbus Dispatch* on March 18, 2008, the day the Buckeyes played a game in the National Invitational Tournament, the consolation prize in big-time college basketball.

I told him at the beginning of the interview that his dad was my doctor when I was fifteen, and I thanked him for taking the time to talk to me. At some point in the interview, I asked him if, as a kid, he knew anything about what his father did for a living. "I know he was a doctor," Kosta said. "I think he did surgeries and stuff."

When he said that, I realized Kosta might not know exactly what his dad did at work. But then again, what nine-year-old does, especially when that father is a pediatric oncologist? I felt guilty. I was here on the grounds that I was doing a story on what it was like for Kosta to grow up without a father, but I really wanted him to tell me everything he knew about his father. I wanted to know more about my doctor, about the man who saved my life, and I wanted to tell someone who knew Dr. Koufos, who loved him, that I would never forget him.

"Well," I said, "he treated kids who had cancer, developed their treatment plans and stuff."

What I wanted to say, what I should have said was "He saved lives. He saved my life."

I must have asked what it was like for him, as a nine-year-old, to see his father become sick.

"I thought it was like any other sickness—he would get over it," Kosta said.

I asked him how memories of his father have impacted him as a college basketball player. He mentioned the fact that his dad kept going to work at the hospital, kept treating patients, kept trying to save lives, even as he was losing his own.

"It just makes me want to work harder at what I do," he said.

I asked him what was going through his mind when his dad died.

"I didn't know what was happening at the time," he said. "It didn't hit me until I saw him in the casket. Seeing his body, I just realized: this is real."

Kosta was every bit as quiet and polite as I had been told he would be. Toward the end of our time, most of the team was on the court shooting, and I could see Kosta's eyes darting their way, wondering when he could escape. I could tell he was the type of man who would not cut the interview short, would not leave even if he wanted to, because he was respectful, because he wanted to answer every single question. In that way, he was exactly like his father. In fact, he reminded me of my doctor so much—not just in his refusal to leave before I was satisfied, but in the way the words came out of his mouth, in the way his eyes looked as he thought about his answers, in the calmness of his voice. I could tell that Kosta would sit there and answer my questions, all the way through practice, if he felt that would be helpful, but I wasn't going to do that to him. He gave me his mother's phone number, and I thanked him for his time and wished him luck with the rest of the season, and I left the arena.

I started driving back to the *Dispatch* when I saw a small pavilion on the banks of the Olentangy River, right across a four-lane boulevard from the arena. I wasn't quite ready to head back to the office because I needed to process the interview, to think about how Kosta's answers could fit into whatever story I was going to write. Even more, I needed to think about why I expected this young man to give me the precious bits of information he had about his dad and how maybe I shouldn't have been the one to write this story after all. I knew deep down that the only reason I pitched the story was to get closer to Kosta, to his family. I needed them to know how much Dr. Koufos had meant to me, and I didn't know any other way to accomplish that.

I pulled into a gravel lot beside the pavilion and walked up to it. A small plaque said it was the Richard and Annette Bloch Cancer Survivors Plaza. Richard Bloch was the cofounder of H&R Block, and he was a fierce crusader for cancer patients. He was also a survivor. He was diagnosed with terminal lung cancer in the late 1970s, yet lived until 2004. Along the way, he founded the RA Bloch Cancer Management Center and the RA Bloch Cancer Support Center. He wrote three books, all cancer-related. He donated the nearly $1.3 million necessary to build the plaza at Ohio State, which thousands pass through on fall Saturdays when the OSU football team plays home games.

The plaza was completed on June 30, 1996. While it was under construction in January of that year, I reached the magical five-year survival mark. Five years is the length of time one needs to live, leukemia-free, to be considered cured of the disease. Five months after it was completed, Dr. Koufos was diagnosed with his cancer.

I pulled up to the front of a nice stone house in a subdivision in Canton. There was a basketball hoop in the driveway, and I found myself wondering, is that the hoop that Dr. Koufos played on with Kosta when he was nine? It looked too new, but maybe? It was a new type of thought for me, one that took Dr. Koufos out of the hospital, away from the cold stethoscopes on my chest and back, and imagined him somewhere else, at home, with a family. That, after all, was why I was here. That was really the point of the story I was working on, even if it wouldn't be the story that would run in the *Dispatch*.

I rang the doorbell and Kathy answered quickly. She was home alone—her children all grown and gone. I walked inside and saw a family picture. In it, Kathy, the kids, and my doctor, her husband and those kids' dad. Then I saw another family picture and then a picture of Dr. Koufos. My heart flooded with warmth when I saw my doctor's face in those pictures. I hadn't realized it, but I had forgotten what he truly looked like. Seeing his image rebooted my memory, replaced that altered image of him with an accurate one.

We spent more than an hour talking at her dining room table, the same table my doctor ate his dinners at. When we talked, it was mostly about Kosta and basketball and his relationship with his dad. We talked about Dr. Koufos's cancer, how he ultimately died, and how Kosta was understandably devastated. I wondered, as we talked about that, whether I should bring up how devastated I was when I heard the news. Should I tell Kathy of the phone call from Nancy? Of how I sat down on my bed and cried like I had never cried before? I didn't tell her this for the same reasons I didn't tell Kosta that his father saved my life. In my mind, I was already writing myself out of this story because I felt I was doing it for the wrong reason, something I think of as absurd ten years later.

"Do you remember the memorial service?" I asked Kathy toward the end of the interview.

"Oh, yes," Kathy said.

"How did that service affect Kosta and the rest of the family?"

Kathy said it was moving, that it was important, especially for Kosta, to learn about the things his father did to help other people. Then Kathy walked over to a cabinet and pulled out a scrapbook. It was the book that everyone wrote messages about Dr. Koufos in at the memorial. There were photos of Dr. Koufos with his patients. (Although not of me. There are no photos of me while I was in the hospital.) There were letters written to Dr. Koufos from patients and their parents. There were letters from parents whose children died, and oftentimes those parents were every bit as thankful for Dr. Koufos as those who survived. That, I think, says something amazing about the type of doctor he was. As we flipped through the pages, I thought back on that night in a way I hadn't in a long time.

Toward the end of the scrapbook was an essay typed on onion-skin paper that was stapled together. My breath caught. I hadn't seen those pages since that night in June 1998, when I stood in front of a crowded auditorium and expressed my sadness and anger at my doctor's death.

We made the drive from Apple Creek to Akron, mostly in silence that evening. The same roads, the same route that Mom and I had driven more than a hundred times (and probably triple that for Mom alone) rushed past. This time we had a third person in the car, and that person was Alyssa. She was my girlfriend at the time, but she would soon be my fiancé, my wife, and the mother of our children. We were heading to Akron Children's Hospital for a memorial service to remember Dr. Koufos. She had never met Dr. Koufos and was curious to know about him. Mom knew Dr. Koufos as well as any parent who would be in that auditorium, I imagined, and revered him more than probably any other human being in the world. I carried with me five pages of writing I had done the week he died, and I intended to read it at the service.

I had spent the last year of my undergraduate college life writing about being sick. It was, for the most part, the first time that I had owned up to the fact that I was a different person, that I was indeed different from everyone else around me, that I looked at life through a lens that had been shaped by an event that nearly killed me.

I wrote papers in philosophy classes that argued against C. S. Lewis's claim that pain was good because it was God's megaphone letting us know that something was wrong, and wrestled with the fact that, for the first time in my life, I wasn't sure there was a god. I wrote about Melissa, mostly, and she was my example to prove that god didn't exist, or that he at least didn't care. I wrote English essays that started exploring exactly how I viewed life now, and how that was different from before I was sick. And I started writing more creative works, stuff that would have been called memoir had I known what memoir was, where I replayed the scenes from what at that point was nearly seven years in the past.

When Dr. Koufos died, it sent me deeper into a search for meaning, and it unleashed a rage at a god I was now sure didn't hear our prayers.

The auditorium at Akron Children's Hospital was packed, and yet people kept streaming in, standing at the back and lining the aisles. Kathy Koufos sat with her three children in the front of the auditorium. The hospital chaplain, Dan Grossoehme, welcomed everyone to the event and talked about how Dr. Koufos was always smiling.

"He was the most gentle and gentlemanly person I've ever known," Grossoehme said. "He talked like a person, not a doctor. He understood what it meant to be a healer."

Grossoehme opened the microphone up to anyone who wanted to say something about Dr. Alex Koufos. This is when the stories started flowing, about how he took a crib to the home of a patient who had sickle cell anemia and assembled it on a Saturday afternoon, about how he bought and delivered a washer and drier to a family, couches to others. He bought clothes and Christmas gifts. This is when a mom wept as she told the story of Dr. Koufos driving to her house as her child lay dying, as he sat and talked with her. This is when a nurse told a story about the time she walked into a room in the outpatient clinic at 6 a.m. to prepare for the start of the day and startled a sleeping Dr. Koufos, who had spent the night in the hospital because one of his patients kept getting sicker and sicker and he needed to be there, to be close, to intervene if the moment warranted it or to comfort if it got worse.

The only person who knew that he had done any of the philanthropic work was Kathy. The nurses didn't know. The other doctors didn't know it. The staff didn't know. And as the stories added up, a fuller picture of the man developed. He cared about everyone he came into contact with; for anyone who faced any danger, he did whatever he could to make them safer.

At one point, a man named John Wood stood up and talked about how Dr. Koufos had saved his daughter's life. He looked at the Koufos children and said their father was a hero.

"Every kid in this room whose life was saved by Alex Koufos, please stand and come forward," Wood said.

Twelve of us stood up.

At some point in the evening, I walked to the front of the room. I had the essay in my hands. I looked at Kathy and her children and started to read. At the time, I knew nothing of Dr. Koufos's personal life or heritage. I didn't know he was Greek (I wasn't smart enough at the time to recognize his name as being Greek), and yet I described him as looking like someone who had just stepped off a boat that had come from the Mediterranean. I read about how tender he was when he visited me. I read about how he often told me my heart was strong. And then I railed against the seemingly unfair way in which he was taken from us.

"I tried to sort through my mind why this would happen to someone who did everything in his power to stop the rage of a disease that took his life," I read to that bursting auditorium. "It didn't seem fair. It wasn't fair."

I finished the piece with this: "And so I cried. I cried because Dr. Koufos wasn't my doctor anymore. I cried because cancer had taken the life of another person whom I cared about. I cried because I never went back to the clinic to go over my records with Dr. Koufos again. I cried because I survived. I cried because Dr. Koufos didn't. I cried because God isn't fair."

In Kathy's house, in the house Dr. Koufos lived in, watched TV in, played with his kids in, I leafed through that essay and cringed at the writing. I was so angry then. But talking with Kosta and Kathy had started to soothe that anger. Knowing more about him, hearing stories about him, brought him back to me in a way I didn't realize could happen.

I told Kathy I had a son. He was three years old, had bright red hair. He was smart. His name was Emery, I told her, which came from my family; it was my great-grandparents' last name. But it was his middle name that I really wanted to tell Kathy about.

"His middle name is Alexander," I said.

That way, he's got part of my doctor's name in his.

Kathy looked like she was blinking back tears.

"That's sweet," she said. "Thank you."

CHAPTER 18

Another Call

Road to Remission is in the closet in the living room of my house in Connecticut. I've had it for nearly twenty-four years now and only played it twice, and one of those times was when we made the video segment. It's moved with my wife and me from apartment to apartment, from city to city, from state to state. It has resided in closets in Wooster, Ohio; Ashland, Ohio; Columbus, Ohio; Wilmington, North Carolina; West Salem, Ohio; and now Newtown, Connecticut. Every time we've moved, I have pulled the game down out of its hiding space and put it in a box, and taken it with me.

I keep it more to remember the names on the box, the kids who worked on it, the kids who didn't survive. But I've thought about Tim and Michael Gray, the two who, when combined with me, made up the three who lived. I didn't know Michael very well and had only met him a time or two. He was younger and from Orrville, like Janet. We never really crossed paths, though, aside from our name appearing on a cardboard box together.

But I think about Tim quite a bit. I often wondered what he was doing in life. Where was he living? Was he married? Did he have kids? What did he tell his kids when they asked about his illness?

I've done some Google searches to see if I could find more out about Tim, but all that comes back are the Associated Press stories about the game. I've searched on Facebook, but there are far too many Tim Snyders on Facebook for me to try and narrow the search. So I go back to just wondering about him, and who he has become.

In 2008, when we lived in Columbus, my son Emery, who was four years old at the time, spotted Road to Remission as it sat on the floor in our basement. Alyssa had been cleaning out and organizing our laundry room, where the game had been sitting on a top shelf, forgotten since the day we moved in. Emery immediately wanted to play the game. It looked like great fun, what with all the colors on the box. Inside, there were four game pieces that were still sealed in plastic. I had never taken them out. I set up the board and figured I'd let Emery draw the cards and I would read them. He wouldn't understand any of it, but he would have fun just moving the pieces back and forth.

I've long known that I would one day have to tell my kids about my illness, about how I nearly died. But I didn't imagine doing it when Emery was four. I couldn't imagine telling my son that his dad was not, indeed, invincible, or that little kids sometimes get sick for no reason at all and that sometimes they die. I didn't want to tell him this right now, and so I figured I would keep things generic, vague.

I drew cards and read them and moved our pieces back and forth. As I read the cards to him, I wondered, did I write that one? Or was it someone else? And if so, who? Was it Shelby or Laura Jo? Was it Tim?

After about fifteen minutes, Emery said he was tired of moving his piece backwards. He asked me to just read the good cards, and I did, all the while imagining how wonderful it would have been if all of us whose names were on that game box, but especially those who didn't live, would have only had to live the good cards. They never would have relapsed. They never would have wasted away. They never would have been the patient from the card "Another patient you know dies."

By 2014, I had been thinking about Tim a great deal. I had started running, and found that when I ran, I often thought about the people I knew when I was sick. And for a while, I was stuck on Tim. I wanted to write about *Road To Remission*, but I felt like any piece on the game needed to be accompanied with an interview with Tim. One day, after another failed Google search, I called Pam and left a voicemail.

"I have a question for you," I said in the message.

She called back a few days later. I was in a committee meeting at Ashland University, where I was a journalism professor, teaching alongside some of the professors who had put up with me during my horrific freshman year. I stepped out of the conference room and into the hallway and answered my phone.

Pam and I chatted for a few minutes. She asked how I was feeling, how my family was. She asked how my mom was, as she always did whenever I talked to her. Then I told her why I called.

"I'm writing about *Road To Remission*," I said, "and I was wondering if you knew what Tim is doing in life right now."

There was silence for what seemed like forever on the other end, and I knew somehow exactly what was coming.

"Oh, Matt," Pam said. "I thought you knew."

"Tim often worries that his cancer will come back, even though it's now in remission."

That was a line from the end of the video segment we made for *Road To Remission* back in the summer of 1992. Tim's worries ultimately came true. He finished high school at Western Reserve Academy in Hudson, Ohio, where he was on the swim team. Then he went to Miami (Ohio) University. He joined a fraternity, but like Melissa, he couldn't finish his first year of college. A new tumor appeared on his hip. Surgeons removed that tumor, and he underwent more chemotherapy. He got a job at a bank and waited to go back to school. But then a tumor appeared on top of his head, then on the nerve in his eye. Eventually, the tumors spread everywhere.

He died on October 24, 1997, more than four and a half years after appearing on national television, one day before the fifth anniversary of Todd's death, and just two months before I saw Dr. Koufos for the last time.

CHAPTER 19

Running With Ghosts

I started running in late August 2012, after having spent the previous twenty years making fun of runners, including my brother Jim, who by that time, had already run two marathons after being a state championship qualifier in both cross country and track and field. I never thought I would start running, then, but when I saw vacation photos of me without a shirt at Myrtle Beach, I wondered who is that whale? I looked so large in the photos that I was shocked. I hadn't stepped on a scale in a long time, but I went upstairs in our house and weighed myself. I weighed more than two hundred pounds.

I wondered how I might be able to lose weight. I tried riding my bike, but my bike was crappy and I hated sitting on that uncomfortable seat. I could join a gym, I thought, but they were so expensive. Even the Ashland University Recreation Center was out of the question, moneywise, because it didn't give discounts to employees, and we were barely scraping by as it was. The most affordable thing to do, I thought, was just run. All I needed was a pair of shoes. So one day, I just took off down the road. It was a mile-and-a-quarter to the interstate from my house in rural Ohio, and so I took off. I barely made it to the interstate and thought I was going to die. I turned around and walked home.

I did that every day, or mostly every day, for a couple weeks. While I ran, I listened to music on my iPhone: the sounds of the 1980s metal band Savatage, the Barenaked Ladies, and Michael Jackson doing the same thing Bon Jovi did for me during spinal taps—taking my mind away from the pain I was feeling. Eventually, we bought a treadmill for the house, and when it got cold, and I found myself on that machine just about every morning. In less than a month, I ran 4.5 miles without stopping on the treadmill. In November, on my birthday, I stayed on that treadmill for ninety minutes and covered six miles. Then I went upstairs and weighed myself. I weighed 180 pounds. I'd lost just about twenty pounds in three months. The last time I shed weight at that rate, I had been lying in a hospital bed, fighting for my life.

I ran a half-marathon on October 6, 2013, in Cleveland. I ran for Team In Training, a major fundraising operation for the Leukemia and Lymphoma Society. I raised about $1,200 and finished the half-marathon in two hours and eighteen minutes. As I pushed through the final mile, I saw Alyssa, the kids, and my mom standing on the side of the road, holding a huge sign that said "Matt Tullis is one tough cookie!" That gave me the energy to push to the finish. The race was brutal. It was hot and humid and I still didn't know what I was doing as a runner, but I learned one thing in the race. I could run without music now, at least if I was outside.

I spent that winter on the treadmill again, listening to whatever I had in iTunes, but also to Spotify. At one point, I started listening to Bon Jovi's *Blaze of Glory*, the album I listened to when Dr. Koufos was crouching behind me and sliding a huge needle into my back. I was struck by how many of the songs on that album were about dying young and thought maybe I should have picked different music for my time in the hospital.

When it warmed up the next spring, I ran outside again. In June, I went for a run without my iPhone, which meant I had no music. I opted instead for the stillness that my mind could reach when the only sensations entering my body were the sights of cornfields and ribbons of asphalt, and the sounds of the wind rustling the tall grasses in the ditches, and my syncopated breathing.

One day, I was running and my thoughts drifted to Janet. I felt like she was just off my left shoulder as we ran on a rural road in Wayne County, Ohio. I had run with her before, but never had I felt her presence so strongly. On this day, I could almost see her, a lithe woman in her forties with brown hair. I had been running this route—an out-and-back, five-and-a-quarter-mile route—at least once a week for about a month. On this run, I was feeling good, running miles under nine minutes, and Janet was keeping up with me, was pushing me. As we passed the three-mile mark, a thought, or more like a sound, entered my brain.

Creech.

I thought about that word, that sound, and tried to place it. I said it out loud. I wondered where I had heard it before. I was thirty-nine years old at the time and had come across many sounds and words in my life as a newspaper reporter, and then later, a college professor. But this word, this sound, I couldn't place it.

"Creech."

I said the word out loud again, and once it escaped my lips, I knew exactly what it was. It was the last name of the woman who was running with me, a name I had been trying to think of for a very long time. For a while, I had envisioned reaching out to her family and letting them know how important she was to me, that I think about her all the time. But I could never do that, because I couldn't remember her last name. Until now.

The more I ran without music blaring in my ears, the more I thought about those who didn't make it. I could feel them running beside me whenever I went out. They pushed me to keep going when I got tired, and cheered me when I ran well.

I thought of Dr. Koufos and Melissa a lot. I thought of Todd hobbling beside me. It was on these early runs that I started thinking about *Road To Remission* and Tim, which resulted in my finding out that he was very much a ghost like the others. I talked with the ghosts as I covered mile after mile. They asked me what I was doing, why I was running. Dr. Koufos asked me how I was feeling and told me my heart was strong.

The road became my sanctuary, the place where I could commune with the dead, think about them, keep them alive somehow, at least in my brain. Remembering Janet's last name pushed me to write the essay titled "The Ghosts I Run With," and it was published and a lot of people read the piece.

A couple of hours after that essay went live online, on April 15, 2015, I received a text message from Kathy, a family friend my wife had met in college and whom we frequently got together with so our kids could play. Kathy grew up in Orrville. She grew up close to Viking Street. She told me one of her best friends in elementary school lived on Viking Street. This friend's mom was named Janet. She had been a nurse and had died in the 1990s.

"Do you think it's her mom?" she asked.

Later that day, I received a message on Facebook from Kathy's friend, Vanessa Corinealdi.

"I just read your post about the ghost you run with," she wrote. "The woman you're discussing is my mother. Thought I would reach out to u! Loved the article!! I am a nurse now too because of her."

Kathy had sent my essay to Vanessa, who read it and then sent it to her brothers and everyone else in her family. She said that Janet, her mom, was her best friend, and that losing her at such a young age was incredibly hard.

"It's nice to hear that somebody else appreciates her," she said. "We all miss her so. It is nice to hear from someone whose life she touched."

The next day, Vanessa emailed me something that Janet wrote in June 1994, just two months before she died. The piece is titled "The Stranger Within" and is about the cancer that was taking her life. She writes, in just about 250 words, the things I have been thinking about for a lifetime—from the unbearable pain to a peaceful silence. It's an introspection into her own life at a time when it was waning.

"I had a good life," she wrote. "Not without care or trouble. But all in all, a good life and full life. Because of the stranger, my thoughts and goals changed from vacations, career, retirement planning, to family and friends. I enjoyed the silence of the stranger. But life was different."

Life was different. It was the same thing Dr. Koufos had told me in 1997, three years after Janet wrote this. It changes you. Cancer changes you. The realization that you could die, that you will die, and possibly soon, changes you in ways that you cannot imagine, until it happens. Janet knew this. Dr. Koufos knew this. Melissa knew this. Deep down, I knew this. But for much of my life, I had a hard time processing exactly what that change meant.

"I am once again enjoying the silence," Janet wrote. "My days are dotted with slight disappointments and nuisances but, oh the joys. I know every crease on my wonderful husband's face. I know the pleasure of a quiet conversation with my sons or daughter. I know every bump and irregularity in my yard where I watch the animals play. I know the joy of a call or a visit from family or friend. But most of all I know God's peace. Only he can silence the stranger within."

By the time I read Janet's writing, I had long since stopped believing in God, let alone with the thought that he would intervene in anyone's life. I had such a hard time believing in a benevolent figure who was just, but who also put people like Janet, Dr. Koufos, and all of my other ghosts through the pain they went through. I had, at one point, become one of those atheists who derided those who believed in God, if not publically, then certainly within my own mind. I would think to myself, you know nothing. You're foolish to believe in something like that. If you had lived my life . . .

But here was Janet, who had, in some way, lived my life. Or something similar. She had gotten to know dozens of kids who ultimately died of cancer. Then she found herself dying of the same disease she had helped treat, and she knew she was dying. She knew the end was near. When she wrote that only God could silence the stranger within, the silencing part was her own death. I couldn't understand that feeling, that belief, but I also didn't think Janet was wrong to believe what she believed near the end, and I'm happy she had that faith.

I wrote in that essay that Janet had breast cancer. I was wrong. I don't know how or why I thought she had breast cancer, other than that was just the most common form of cancer and that somehow made sense in my mind. I got an email from Janet's older sister, Rhonda, and she corrected me, pointing out that Janet's cancer started in her gall bladder, something rare in someone her age.

"I wanted a rare diamond," Rhonda remembers her sister saying often, "not a rare cancer."

My ghosts had been accompanying me everywhere I went, and not just when I was out running. I was thinking about Dr. Koufos, Janet, Melissa, Todd, Tim, and others all the time. I thought about them when I drove to the Ashland University campus and when I drove into the West Salem IGA store to pick up a few odds and ends that we needed to make dinner. I thought of them when I drove my daughter, Lily, to school, and when I picked her up. I thought of them when I sat on my back deck and stared west, watching thunderstorms roll in from more than thirty miles away.

I realized, though, after hearing from Janet's family, that I didn't know that much about my ghosts. When I thought of them, I thought of them in the context of my own illness. I thought of Janet bringing me a sausage biscuit, of Dr. Koufos doing a spinal tap or pressing a cold stethoscope to my chest. I thought of Tim and *Road to Remission* and of Todd falling off a horse. I thought of Melissa walking like a stork. I was just repeating the same stories and thoughts in my head over and over again. But now I felt like I needed to know more. I had to know more because I wanted to make them more real in my mind. I wanted to know as much about my ghosts as I could, and I wanted to make sure any memories I had of them were accurate.

There was, fortunately, one thing about Janet in my essay that was right in ways I could never have imagined. I took a quick breath when I read it in her own writing.

"I once ran," Janet wrote in the first paragraph of her piece. "Daily running. Running to relieve the stress of a busy life and work. Running to strengthen my body and enjoy our world."

I imagined Janet going home and running through the streets of Orrville after a day spent being my nurse. Maybe she ran the day she had to come to room 462 eighteen times in eight hours, that day when I stood up and blood just started dripping down my chest, out of my central line. Maybe she ran after that shift when I had an allergic reaction to the L-asparginase shot in my thigh, and she had to rush out and get me Benedryl. Maybe she ran the day that she found out I had been moved to intensive care. I can see her moving through the streets, past Crown Hill Cemetery in Orrville, where I've watched the city's fireworks, on down past Orr Park, where I played high school baseball, and then later, slow-pitch softball. Maybe she even ran out past McDonald's, where she would stop the next morning to pick up a sausage biscuit for me.

I didn't, of course, know then that Janet was a runner. But she was the first person I had ever imagined running beside me when I was out on the road. Now, she was the first one to give me a bit of information. It seemed perfect that she was a runner, like this puzzle that was my life was starting to fit together, to make some sense.

Later that summer, I was sitting in the basement living room of Denny Forrer, Janet's husband. After "The Ghosts I Run With" was published, Denny's daughter, and subsequently Janet's stepdaughter, contacted me. Christine Domer was a seventh-grade teacher in Orrville schools, and her students had just read a book about a boy with leukemia. She had read my piece, she said, and was moved by the idea that someone else who they didn't know still thought about Janet on a regular basis. She asked me if I would come talk to the seventh-graders in the school about what it was like to have leukemia and to survive.

I did, of course, and afterward I asked Christine if she thought her dad would ever want to talk to me about Janet.

"I'll ask him," she said, before adding that he was still broken up about Janet's death, even though it had been more than twenty years.

Ultimately, Denny agreed to meet with me. Denny no longer lives on Viking Street. After he retired from the city of Orrville, he moved into a condo on the other side of town. When I got to his place, he had a bunch of pictures of Janet spread out on an ottoman, photos of them on vacation in the Caribbean and photos of her just sitting in their house. For both Janet and Denny, their marriage was a second chance. They had both been married before, and both had children from those relationships. Denny met Janet at a dance in Akron for single parents. He was immediately smitten with her. He was taken aback by her kindness and gentleness.

They created a wonderful family on Viking Street. Janet would go to work at the hospital and then come home and go running or sit on the patio and watch the cows in the field behind their house. She spent a great deal of time with the kids. She and Denny took great vacations to warm, sunny places where they went scuba diving.

They were together for only about five or six years before Janet got sick. Janet fought that stranger, the cancer that invaded her body, as best she could. She got the best medical treatment available. She kept working on the floor at Akron Children's, taking care of patients. Hospital administrators told her she needed to wear a wig because her not having hair might scare patients, but like Dr. Koufos in his refusal to wear a tie or a lab coat, Janet said no, that a wig would not make her a better nurse. Instead, she wore a bandana over her bald head.

"She didn't like the wig because it itched," said Theresa, my nurse from the fourth floor, as well as one of Janet's best friends. "She fought long and hard. She said, 'Once the kids see me, what's the difference? They'll know this isn't my hair.' She wore the bandanas and that was fine, and she looked absolutely beautiful."

Janet took Christine, who was older than Vanessa, wedding dress shopping, because she knew she would never get the chance to do that with Vanessa. In the end, she spent her final days on her patio, staring out at the cows as they munched on grass and lived their otherwise quiet lives.

I talked with Denny for about an hour. I didn't take many notes, just sat there and listened to him talk about the woman who was the ultimate love of his life. They were perfect for each other, in much the same way that Janet was perfect for the nursing profession. She poured her whole body and soul into her marriage with Denny and into raising the children that they brought together into one family in much the same way she poured herself into taking care of kids like me. It wasn't just a job for her. That's a thought I have long had with regard to Janet and her career as a nurse. Even as a patient, I could tell she was different, different from some of the other women who came into my room and gave me medications and checked my blood pressure. Like Theresa, she was present in a way others weren't, in a way that is hard to put into words. Her humanity was intensified, in much the same way Dr. Koufos's was. And it was evident.

Denny confirmed those thoughts that I had, helped me realize that I wasn't just mythologizing someone who died long before they should have. As we talked about Janet, he wiped away tears. He became choked up several times. He had not gotten over losing her and it had been nearly twenty-one years.

In the spring of 2016, I found myself hanging out at Akron Children's Hospital about once every couple weeks. I was spending a lot of time going over my medical records, building timelines, and trying to decipher Dr. Koufos's handwriting, which sometimes was easy to read and other times was incredibly difficult. I looked at those records in Pam's office, so I got to ask her a lot of questions as well. Some of the questions were medical-related, like "what does 75 percent blast mean in a bone marrow biopsy?" Other questions were about people. Did she know where Todd's parents lived now? Did she remember exactly when Tim died? Where were his parents? Those questions were oftentimes unanswerable. It had all happened so long ago, and so many people, like Pam, had pushed the bad memories out and maintained the memories of those who survived, like me.

One day I went and talked with Theresa. When I was in the hospital, Theresa and Janet were the cochampions in the race to be fifteen-year-old Matt's favorite nurses. Theresa is still at Akron Children's, only now she is the nurse manager for the 5600 floor, which is where today's childhood cancer patients stay.

The day before I talked with Theresa, Akron Children's unveiled a sculpture dedicated to nurse Bonnie Leighley, who worked at the hospital for fifty-one years before dying in 2014. The sculpture was unveiled during National Nurses Week, on Florence Nightingale's birthday, May 12. Theresa said she was in tears when the sculpture was unveiled because she was thinking about Leighley but also about Janet.

"They were talking about Bonnie's legacy here," Theresa said. "There are so many people who have strong legacies, and Janet is one of them. No matter what, she continued to work."

I asked Theresa to tell me a story about Janet as a nurse, one that didn't involve me.

Before Janet got sick, Theresa said, maybe even before I got sick and became one of her patients, she and Theresa were taking care of a parentless toddler who was on dialysis. Janet was taking care of the girl from 7 a.m. to 3 p.m., and Theresa was her nurse from 3 to 11 p.m. Easter was coming up, and Theresa wanted to do something nice for the girl.

"We've got to get her out of here," Theresa told Janet.

The girl was just about to turn three years old and had never really had a home. She went from a medical foster home to the hospital and then to another foster home and back to the hospital. Theresa asked a doctor if she and Janet could take the girl out on a day pass, and he let them. They took her to Belden Village Mall in Canton.

"We had her out for four hours," Theresa said. "We bought her three Easter dresses and hats so she would have some clothes to wear."

She ate pickles and slices of pepperoni, which required dialysis when she got back to the hospital, but that's what the girl wanted, and the doctor told Theresa and Janet to give the girl what she wanted.

What she wanted more than anything, though, was to ride the escalators. They went up and down and up and down, over and over again. They took pictures of her on the escalator, and of her eating salty foods. They gave that girl one of the best days of her life, Theresa said.

I think about Janet on that escalator, going up and then down and then up and then down. I imagine the girl squealing with delight, just as my own kids did the first times they rode an escalator. I remember them begging to go again and again and again, and so we did that too. The simplest things can bring us joy, especially when we are sick, when our lives are threatened, and so when I think of Janet on that escalator, I also think of her going through the drive-through at McDonald's early on a winter morning and ordering a sausage biscuit, not for herself, but for a boy who was lying in a hospital bed, dreading the breakfast tray with soggy bacon and bland oatmal, a boy who needed more than anything else to eat something, anything, to survive the barrage of drugs that were entering his body, a boy who would light up when she walked into his room in just about an hour, and who still lights up when he thinks of her, so many years later.

CHAPTER 20

The Planner

I had a voicemail on my office phone at Ashland University in the fall of 2015.

"This is Mrs. Lanning," the message started out. "I think you wrote about my daughter."

It was incredibly short, void of details. She left her phone number, which I wrote down. I thought for a moment about how I might have written about a Mrs. Lanning's daughter. The most recent thing I had written of any consequence had been my piece, "The Ghosts I Run With." I called Mrs. Lanning, and as soon as she started talking, I knew. The voice, oh the voice. The voice was Melissa's as much as it was anyone else's, all sharp and accented like someone straight off the streets of Boston. I had always known Melissa's last name, but I just didn't put two and two together until this moment. It turns out Louise, which is Mrs. Lanning's first name, didn't read my piece on SB Nation. She saw it when it was reprinted in *Accent*, Ashland University's alumni magazine. The university had asked to rerun the piece because I was a faculty member who also happened to be an alumnus.

A friend of Louise's, who had gone to Ashland University, read the story. She knew about Melissa and did the math with regard to the passage of time and thought that maybe the Melissa in my piece might have been Louise's Melissa. She sent the magazine on to her friend. Louise read the story and had a good inkling that the Melissa I was writing about was her Melissa. There was just one problem.

"My Melissa didn't have leukemia," Louise said on the phone.

That's what I had written in the piece because that's what I remembered. Just like with Janet, I had gotten the type of cancer wrong. This is one thing that has troubled me as I write about being sick—how often my memory is wrong. It's impossible to imagine that, while we were hanging out at Camp CHOPS, Melissa didn't tell me specifically what type of cancer she had. That was the conversation starter in the same way "What's your major?" is in college. So, at one point, I knew that she had rhabdomyosarcoma. But I had let her type of cancer evolve into my type of cancer so we could be more similar, so I could understand why it was I was so wrecked over her death. It wasn't enough for me to just be sad because a friend of mine had died. I needed to tie her death to my own cancer, something I'm only now starting to realize I do, something that is wholly self-centered and absurd.

"The Melissa I wrote about was from Millersburg and had black hair," I said.

"That's her," Louise said.

We talked briefly on the phone. Louise thanked me for writing about her daughter, and I told her I would love to talk with her more about Melissa. I was starting to realize that I knew very little about the people I thought about all the time.

Louise doesn't live in Millersburg anymore. She and her husband Jim divorced after Melissa died. Louise moved about thirty miles north into a condo in a development in Wooster. The first time I met her, we walked to her dining room table and sat down.

"I think I have a picture of you," she said.

Louise had a lot of pictures of Melissa on the table, in much the same way Denny had set out pictures of Janet, and the Koufos house is full of photos of my doctor. There are photos where she is bone thin, wearing sweatshirts that are too big and glasses that take up most of her face. There's a photo of her in a tuxedo with a skirt instead of pants, a hat on top of her bald head, a cane holding her steady, as she gets ready to go to her senior prom, just six months after she found out she had cancer. I find these pictures interesting because there are so few photos of me when I was sick. There's nothing from the hospital, despite the fact I spent nearly ten weeks there. The earliest photo I've been able to find of me postcancer is one at my brother John's birthday party in May, four months after I went into the hospital.

Louise also had photos of Melissa looking completely healthy, young, and vibrant. In some, she looks like she's a middle schooler, in others, a sophomore or junior in high school. In these photos, she's living completely unaware of what is about to happen to her. These are the photos of the

Melissa I never knew, the Melissa who didn't know that she would one day walk like a stork or come to love a camp for kids who had cancer.

Louise did have a photo of me, and it was from Camp CHOPS. There are six of us in the photo—Melissa, Sharon, Kim, me, and two boys I don't know. It's from 1993. Sharon and I are crouched down in the front. I am right in front of Melissa. I'm wearing an old Cubs hat, and my hair is hanging out the back, just like it did before I got sick. I'm wearing glasses, which I had only recently gotten. Melissa is smiling in the photo as well. We all are smiling, actually, unlike the photo from the year before, in the hot air balloon, when we all looked stone-faced at the camera.

I had never seen this photo, hadn't even remembered posing for it. Louise said she would make me a copy, and I thanked her.

"You know," I said. "I kind of had a crush on Melissa."

"Oh yeah?" Louise said. "She came home from camp once and said there's this boy who likes her."

"He's way too young," Melissa said to her mom.

I laughed, but actually liked the fact Melissa may have noticed how badly I wanted to spend time with her.

I met with Louise a couple times. And then, I showed up one day and Jim Lanning, Melissa's dad, was there as well. The dining and living rooms of Louise's condo are connected in an open arrangement, and while she sat on a chair at the table, Jim sat in a chair that was on the other side of the room, near a window that was pouring in sunlight. We talked about Dr. Koufos, and Louise asked me if I knew anything about his wife, whether she was still living in the area. I told them that Kathy Koufos still lived in the same house that she and Dr. Koufos lived in, and that she had told me she would never sell it because she can still feel his presence there. Louise said that her brother had just lost his wife—he just woke up one morning and she had died in the night. They owned a huge Victorian home, but he would also never move for the same reason.

Eventually, we started talking about Melissa, but as we do, I'm cognizant of the fact we are talking about her in a place where she had never been. Aside from the photos, Melissa does not have a presence here. In fact, when Melissa was alive, the development that is now home to Louise's condo was a cornfield on the outskirts of Wooster. It was not a place she would have ever been, ever had a presence to attach to. Both Louise and Jim had moved on, at least as far as place goes. But their memories of their daughter were still strong. She was still present in their lives, and I wanted her to be more present in mine, to understand more of who she was.

This is who Melissa was:

She was a girl, who, in the third grade, ran for student council but didn't get a single vote, not even from herself. Another time, she wrote a play for class, but nobody wanted to be in it with her.

She was bossy, a spark plug, a girl who was going to do what she was going to do. That may be why nobody voted for her, and why nobody wanted to be in her play. But even though those things tore her up at the time, they didn't change who she was, because she wasn't going to change for anybody.

When she played soccer as a kid, she had to be put on a different team than her brother Jimmy because during the game she would just stand there and tell Jimmy what he should have been doing.

She loved to play poker.

Wishes Can Happen gave her money for a car, and her brother-in-law spent two months customizing it. She called the car Mel. I knew she had this awesome car because I rode in it once. I didn't know that she drove it for less than two months—including the day she drove from Millersburg to Apple Creek to pick me up on our way to Cleveland, to hang out with our Camp CHOPS friends—because one day, she was driving through Millersburg and an elderly woman pulled out in front of her and T-boned that beautiful white car. The insurance wouldn't pay to cover the extensive customizations, and yet Melissa refused to even consider suing the older woman. She ended up driving a car that was similar, but was no Mel. But it was the right thing to do, and she did it.

Melissa's best friend in the world was a girl named Mary Ann. Mary Ann lived in Massachusetts, across the street from Louise's sister. Melissa would go up to Massachusetts and stay with her aunt for weeks on end, and just spend all of that time hanging out with Mary Ann. At one point, she asked her mother if she could go to high school in Massachusetts because that's where she felt like she belonged, but Louise wouldn't let her, couldn't imagine living in Millersburg without her.

She worked as a cashier at Rhode's IGA in Millersburg while in high school.

Melissa was the type who would stay up late but still wake up early and help everyone get ready for the day.

She collected Barbie dolls, but refused to take them out of the box.

Melissa was a planner. Even from a hospital bed, she insisted on planning birthday parties for her parents. During her first stay at Akron Children's, she planned Jim's fiftieth birthday party and then got a day pass to go home for the party she had planned.

The first time she received chemotherapy, she looked at Jim after about an hour of a continuous IV drip and said, "I think I'm going to be all right, Papa. I don't feel anything yet." An hour later she said, "Papa, I think I'm going to be sick."

Melissa loved to sing and dance. She was in the choir. She loved sports, but wasn't any good at them.

She was tough as nails and hot as fire. You couldn't tell her no. She was so tough that Jim nicknamed her Ryu (pronounced Roo). It doesn't sound like such a tough nickname, but Jim at the time had been studying the form of martial arts known as Isshin-ryu, which is a particularly hard and tough form of karate. The term also means wholehearted and complete, which would have also suited Melissa as well.

She went to college for one year—at the Ohio University branch in Zanesville. This happened in the fall after I met Melissa for the first time at Camp CHOPS, the weekend we spent a few minutes standing in a hot air balloon for a picture and a few hours playing euchre, the same weekend Todd fell off a horse and I freaked out. During this year of college, she took courses like Spanish, Japanese, and international business. She got all As, Jim said. She was going to do amazing things.

As Louise and Jim tell these stories about their daughter, stories I never knew or maybe knew at one point and then forgot, tears came to their eyes and mine, and their throats caught. Then they told me about when her cancer came back.

Before finals of her last quarter at OU in June 1993, a week or two after her trip to Camp CHOPS, she realized she was sick again.

"I just feel terrible, Mom," she told Louise over the phone from her dorm room.

She came home and went to the doctor. The cancer had come back.

Melissa broke down once she was back in the hospital. She refused to talk to anybody. She yelled at Louise, "Get out! Get out! I don't want you here!" She said, "Mom, I want you to go!" She said, "I hope that after I'm dead you enjoy spending the insurance money and think about me when you do!"

She refused to talk to Jim for three months.

She was angry, at her parents, at herself, at the world, maybe even at God. And then she came around, she felt guilty and ashamed of the things she said to Louise and the things she refused to say to Jim.

"No one knows how much that rips my heart out to think about!" Melissa wrote in her diary. "Not only that, but how I treated Mom and Dad too, then and lately."

On a drive home from the clinic one day, after Melissa had received another heavy dose of chemotherapy, she lay across the back seat of Jim's car. She was talking to him by this point, and she asked him a question he can't repeat without breaking down in tears.

"Papa, I know I'm going to die," he remembers her saying. "Do you know when that's going to happen?"

He told her only God knew when it was going happen.

She spent the next eighteen months planning her own funeral. She called the preacher and told him that his sermon was going to focus on the road to salvation in the New Testament book of Romans. She decided that the memorial service was going to open with Michael Jackson's "Gone Too Soon," and that the opening hymn was going to be "Crown Him With Many Crowns," but only the first and third stanzas. She decided that Pastor Dave Truit and Mary Ann Denson would read Isaiah 40:28–31, Psalm 23:1–6 and John 14:1–6. She decided that the gospel reading and homily would be John 3:16–18 and Matthew 11:28–30, and would also include St. Francis's poem "Sister Death." She decided the congregation would sing "Amazing Grace" and "Old Rugged Cross," and that the service would end with the hymn "He Lives."

She was a girl and then a woman who was in complete control, even when she wasn't.

CHAPTER 21

The Finest Physician

There was a photo posted in the late winter of 2016 on Facebook and Twitter by Akron Children's Hospital that made me do a double take. In the photo, a very tall young man stood with four nurses from the Hematology and Oncology clinic. I recognized two of the nurses immediately. They were Pam and Char, another nurse who often took care of me when I was receiving chemotherapy on an outpatient basis. I recognized the young man as well. At seven feet tall, Kosta Koufos is hard not to recognize. He only played college basketball at The Ohio State University for one year before declaring for the 2008 National Basketball Association draft. He was picked in the first round that year. Now he's on the Sacramento Kings. I looked at that photo longer than I normally would have, though, because I saw Dr. Koufos in Kosta. Maybe it was the juxtaposition with nurses I knew from my days as a patient, but I really could see Dr. Koufos looking out from that photo.

Kosta was in Akron at the hospital on a day during the NBA's All-Star break. It was his first trip home to Canton since the summer before. He had been doing some outreach with Akron Children's, and was setting up a foundation for children with cancer in his father's name. This was one of his first trips back to the hospital that his dad used to bring him to for weekend rounds. Kosta had avoided the hospital because it reminded him so much of the fact his dad was gone. He spent the day hearing stories about Dr. Koufos and how much fun he had as a doctor, as well as how hard he worked. Kosta has always held his dad up as a model for work ethic, a man who kept working even after he was given a death sentence.

The photo left me thinking of my doctor the rest of the day. I knew more about him than I did just about any of the other ghosts, partly because of the story I wrote on Kosta when he was in college. I also spent more time with Dr. Koufos than any of my other ghosts. I've been lucky enough to have lunch with Kosta one day after "The Ghosts I Run With" was published and then talk again with him and his mom on the phone. I've done more research into Dr. Koufos than anyone else because I think about him all the time. I want others to know about him, how special he was, how instrumental he was, not just in my life, but in so many others'.

Alex Koufos was born in Canton, Ohio, in 1952. His parents' families were from Corinth, Greece, but the Koufos clan had been in America for many decades. Alex went to Canton's McKinley High School, and when school was not in session, he bagged groceries at Fishers grocery store, earning money to help his family. Later, when he had enrolled at Akron University and then The Ohio State University, he continued to work at Fishers during school breaks to help with his tuition bills. He stayed in Columbus after earning his undergraduate degree, entering OSU's School of Medicine. The three-year residency program at Ohio State had Alex rotating through different areas of specialty, but it was in hematology and oncology that he found his passion.

He completed an internship at Cincinnati Children's Hospital, where he treated patients and began his research into developing a treatment for children with soft tissue sarcoma, a fairly rare form of cancer that forms in muscles, fat, tendons, and blood vessels. He discovered that chromosomal gene injuries or mutations occur in this kind of tumor, which resulted in his publishing a paper in *Nature* in 1985. That was just one of his many scientific publications.

It was while he was a medical student at Ohio State that Alex met Kathy. She was born in Greece, but moved with her family to Australia when she was seven years old, and then later to Canton after that. Alex came home for a weekend and went to a big, Greek community picnic at the end of August. Kathy, who had just graduated from Malone College in Canton, said her uncle and Alex's uncle wanted to make sure the two met each other at this picnic. "I was like, I'm not going to meet anyone," Kathy said. But somehow they ended up sitting next to each other, and they started talking.

"I knew from the very beginning when I met him," Kathy said. That was the type of impact he had on her. And she had an impact on him. "I loved his intelligence. I loved his humility. I loved the fact that he could talk about so many different things and he was so well versed in things, and I was impressed that he had read philosophy and Plato and Socrates."

After a couple of dates, Kathy knew she would marry Alex Koufos. They were engaged by December and married by the following July.

Once Alex's fellowship was up in Cincinnati, Alex and Kathy decided to move to Canada, where he would continue his research at the Ludwig Cancer Institute in Montreal. He worked in a lab as a research scientist for seven years, but realized he missed working with patients. He was eager to get back to a clinic setting, and getting a Canadian license was difficult, so the Koufos family, now consisting of son Vasilious and daughter Maria, started looking to move back to Ohio.

Dr. Frederick Ruymann, who was head of the Hematology and Oncology Department at Columbus Children's Hospital at the time, wanted him to come to Columbus. But as the family was looking for a place to land in Ohio, Alex's father passed away. Feeling as though he needed to be near his mother, he moved the family back to Canton. Around the same time, the hematology and oncology clinic at Akron Children's Hospital, just a thirty-minute commute from his and Kathy's hometown, was looking for a pediatric oncologist. Alex took the job. That was in 1989. Kosta was born shortly after the move. Two years after taking the job in Akron, Dr. Koufos met a very sick boy from Apple Creek.

I have, over the two decades that have passed since Dr. Koufos died, mythologized the man in my mind. He has reached the level of sainthood as I spend moments every single day thinking about him and how he saved my life. Surely, if I had been assigned to another doctor, the result may have been the same, but he was so calm, so caring, so willing to give of his own personal time, that he made us—my parents and I—feel like I was the only person he was taking care of, and that played a huge role in my survival. Would other doctors have done what he did? I saw dozens of other doctors while I was in Akron, some of them incredibly nice but hurried, some of them harsh and of the asshole variety. Comparing them all with Dr. Koufos just makes him that much more memorable and perfect.

In my last year as a full-time newspaper reporter, I started writing feature obituaries. I scanned the paid obits in the day's paper, looking for someone, a normal person, who should have their life story told. Then I reached out to the family and asked if they would talk to me. They invariably said yes they would, and I went to their homes, the ones they shared with the person who had died, and we talked for several hours about that person's life. One thing I always asked during these meetings was for the loved ones to tell me something about the dead person that drove them crazy, that they hated, that they couldn't stand. We have a tendency to lionize the dead, to not want to say anything bad about someone who has passed on. That elevates everyone to sainthood. Everyone is perfect when we talk about them that way, which makes them less human because nobody is perfect. Those families always come up with something, and when they do, they laugh. One old woman whose husband had just died told me that he never let her pick the radio station in the car. The father of a twenty-five-year-old woman who was killed in a car crash on Thanksgiving told me how he couldn't stand his daughter's morbid sense of humor.

I've asked this same question to every person I've interviewed about Dr. Koufos, and nobody can answer it. They can't think of anything about Dr. Alex Koufos that annoyed them or drove them crazy or even just made them think, *I wish he wouldn't do that.* The best his wife can come up with is the fact he was overly protective. Basically, he cared too much.

I try to answer this question myself, and I settle on the fact he ordered a feeding tube to be placed in my stomach on January 21, 1991, because I had lost more than twenty pounds in my first two weeks in the hospital. My hatred of that episode stemmed from the painful way in which the tube was snaked up my nose and down my throat, the plastic scraping my esophagus, making me choke and gasp for air as one of my favorite nurses encouraged me to take sips of water to help the tube slide down. And even worse; the tube frequently clogged. It had to be replaced at least twice through the same horrible procedure. That was certainly a momentary hatred, one born out of the pain I was feeling as a patient, from my complete feeling of helplessness. But it evaporated the moment the tube was no longer necessary, and it seems trivial now, a quarter-century later, when I realize exactly how important it was that my body get some nutrition to help it in the battle I was fighting.

In Akron, Alex had a reputation as both a brilliant scientist and physician, as well as a person who was respectful of every person he came into contact with. Pam said he was the first doctor she ever worked with who insisted she call him by his first name, and not by Dr. Koufos. "He was the finest physician I have ever worked with," she said. "He was brilliant and so caring."

He traveled to the homes of patients when they were in their final hours so he could help alleviate the anguish the parents were facing. When those dying patients were in the hospital, he spent the night.

Alex won the Golden Apple Teaching Award for teaching residents three years in a row. He didn't wear ties or lab coats because he worried they would scare the little children that he took care of. And he didn't just treat their cancers. He sat down with them and played and drew pictures, whatever those sick little kids wanted to do.

"I loved when Alex had clinic day," Pam said. "We just had a fun day. If you were concerned about something, you could go to him. If you were worried about something, you could go to him."

And so it was, he would walk into my clinic room and tell me he barely graduated from high school when I told him I had a big test coming up, and that everything would work out, no matter how I did on the test. He would talk to Mom like she was the most important person on the planet. He would put his stethoscope to my chest, apologize for its coldness, and then tell me I had a strong heart.

In Akron, and indeed everywhere he worked, Alex worked long hours. He was always looking for new and better treatments. He took medical texts with him on family vacations. While his wife and kids played in the ocean, he sat on the beach, puzzling over a patient or a new chemotherapy protocol while simultaneously worrying that Kathy had taken the kids out too far into the water, that they were going to be sucked away by a rip current.

He'd look up from his book and start waving his hands at Kathy.

"Come back!" he'd shout. "You're too far out!"

Kathy knew what he was saying even if she couldn't hear him over the wind and the waves.

"Wave at your father," she told the kids, laughing. "He's waving to us."

Eventually Kathy and the kids would come back to the beach, and Alex would say, "Didn't you see me motioning to bring them back in? You went too far."

"Oh, I thought you were waving at us," Kathy said.

They'd laugh, even Alex, because it was all right. They were all still safe, collapsed on the sand around him.

Because of his dedication to work, he missed many events in his children's lives. He found ways to get to a basketball game or a music recital, but not nearly as often as he would have liked. But when he was home, he was present, physically and emotionally, for his children. He loved to watch X-Files on Friday nights in the living room, the whole family on the couch, even a young Kosta. He made sure he was home for dinner just about every night. He played basketball with Kosta and listened in disbelief as Vasilious played the piano. Sometimes they would go downstairs and play with the Lionel model train set that was in the basement.

"He had a Lionel layout booklet," Kosta says. "I remember one night we changed the layout eight or nine times, and he asked me which one I liked best."

That's one of Kosta's fondest memories of his dad partly because Alex was sick at the time.

Dr. Koufos became depressed after finding out he had cancer that was basically untreatable and inoperable. He wanted to give up. Perhaps he couldn't take the irony that he, a man who had spent his life battling cancer, now had a type that, for the most part, could not be battled. Perhaps it was the fact that he knew too much. In the beginning, when I got sick, I was too naïve, too dumb, to know that I could die. I didn't know the survival rate for my kind of cancer was hovering between 50 and 60 percent until years later, when I began doing research for my writing. I knew I was sick, but that was it. Dr. Koufos knew everything there was to know about his cancer. While he might not have seen it in one of his childhood patients, he surely ran across it somewhere, in medical school, in his research. For his cancer, the only chance at achieving long-term survival—and this only offered a 15 to 25 percent chance—was surgery to remove the tumor. Unfortunately, he quickly learned that his tumor was inoperable.

The despair, sadness, and anger boiled over when Alex was ready to give up, and he and Kathy had a fight.

"This is not what you would do for any of your patients," Kathy told him. "You would never give up on any of your patients. Don't you dare give up on yourself and us."

Whether it was that talk or something else, Alex began to fight. He and Kathy traveled the country, looking for the best treatment for his cancer. They ended up at the University of Michigan in Ann Arbor, where an aggressive regimen of chemotherapy and radiation would be used to at least try and slow the cancer's growth. It worked, at least as far as keeping it from spreading. Alex and Kathy began exploring the possibility of a liver transplant, but he was turned down in Pittsburgh and at Johns Hopkins Hospital in Baltimore because doctors there still were not sure where the cancer was going. Still, buoyed by the fact the cancer's growth had stopped and he was feeling better, Alex returned to Akron Children's Hospital and started seeing a limited number of patients again. He did that for about a year after his initial diagnosis. For Alex, to take away his life's work was to take away everything, and so he threw himself into his patients.

He had lost a lot of weight from the chemotherapy and radiation, and occasionally, someone who hadn't seen him in a while and who didn't know he had cancer would say, *Wow, you've lost a lot of weight. How'd you do it?*

"Oh, just a new weight-loss plan," he would say, chuckling.

At home, he played with his kids. They played catch and he rebounded basketballs. He listened to music with them. They watched *X-Files* together on the couch in the living room. He fished with his kids in the pond out behind their house. He worried about the safety of his children and about the lives of all the children he had treated.

I saw Dr. Koufos only twice after he was diagnosed with cancer. The last time I saw him before he became a cancer patient was on December 21, 1995. I went on that day for what had become a yearly checkup. After that visit, though, I didn't come back until June 2, 1997, just a few days before Camp CHOPS, at which I would be a full-blown counselor. At that time, I was working at a daily newspaper as an intern after three summers of working in factories. I don't know why I waited eighteen months to see Dr. Koufos again, other than the fact I was told he wasn't seeing patients in December of 1996, when I should have seen him. I have no memory of that first postcancer meeting with him. I don't know what we talked about. I probably told him about my work at the newspaper and about my girlfriend, Alyssa. He probably told me my heart was strong, after pressing a cold stethoscope to my chest.

I would see him again six months later, and that's when he told me life was different now, and that I was one sick cookie. And then I'd never see him again.

I think about that time, the more than two years that Dr. Koufos had cancer, a time in which I saw him only twice, and am filled with regret. I feel as though I should have been there, in some way, to help him the way he helped me. But I also know rationally that I couldn't save him.

Vasilious had a birthday shortly after his father died. For a long time, he and the other kids had wanted a trampoline in the backyard.

"Absolutely not," Alex said. "They're going to injure themselves. The kids are going to have broken bones all the time."

But now, Kathy thought the kids needed something, anything, to lighten the mood. She thought, *Alex, you're not going to like this*, and then she bought a trampoline for Vasilious's birthday. They all worked together to assemble it, and it took all evening. It was after midnight once the trampoline was finally usable, and so the four of them got on and started jumping up and down and up and down and up and down. After a while, once they were out of breath and all jumped out, they lay down on the black canvas of the trampoline and looked up at the stars and started talking about the man they had just lost.

"What would your dad say right now," Kathy asked her kids.

"I can't believe you did this!" one of the kids said.

"Think of all the injuries," someone else said.

"How could you be so careless?!?"

"I'm sorry honey,'" Kathy said to the sky. "But this is something that was needed for all of them to get out of the sadness and the grief. And we laughed and enjoyed it."

Nobody was ever hurt on the trampoline.

"He was always so protective of the kids and always looking after them," Kathy said, and she meant after he had died as well.

I still have dreams where Dr. Koufos shows up and starts asking me how I am doing. I'm always my current age in these dreams, but he is as he was from 1991–93 when I was sick. He asks me how I'm feeling and how school is going. Once I said, "But you're dead, Dr. Koufos," and he chuckled. Once, when I was in grad school, he asked me how my book was coming along. We talked about it, and I told him I wished he could read it someday.

One day in the summer of 2016, I was having lunch with Kosta. He had read "The Ghosts I Run With" and said he wanted to help with the book, to tell me stories about his dad. I told him about the dream, particularly the one from grad school. And I swear he chuckled, just like Dr. Koufos chuckled, and said he dreams of his dad all the time. He said he can still feel him in the house in Canton.

"When I'm working on the train set, I feel like he is there," Kosta said. "His presence is in the house. I truly believe that he is there with us."

Lately, I've felt as though I've abandoned the work that Dr. Koufos did for me. I've been thinking a lot about the time in 2006, when I went back to Akron Children's for a late-effect clinic checkup. Those types of checkups are becoming more popular and important for childhood cancer survivors because there are more of us thanks to the amazing treatments, but also because those treatments are causing issues, sometimes twenty years down the line.

When I went in 2006, though, I went through the motions. In truth, I made that visit because I saw it as being the end of a part of my life (and, truthfully, the end of the book). I would have the checkups, be told I was awesome, and go home, triumphant. And it's true; the echocardiogram and the bone density tests showed that I was doing all right in those areas. But I had other issues, and I ignored them all. I should have been visiting this late-effect clinic once a year, but I never went back to the one in Akron. The only thing I have done is see a dermatologist regularly. I also started exercising by running, but that didn't happen until seven years after that visit to the late-effect clinic. That was the year I became depressed, which ultimately led to testosterone treatments and a partial reassessment of my life. I finally got myself a primary care physician and an endocrinologist. But I still didn't care much for my teeth, apparently, and I didn't care much for the type of food and drink I put in my body. I steadfastly refused sunscreen because of the idiotic claim that "I'm going to get skin cancer anyway," and opted to just keep going under the knife every time a new basal cell appeared. It must have been exasperating to Pam, although she never said anything to me about it.

Ten years after that visit, I moved with my family to Connecticut, and Pam put me in touch with the late-effect clinic at the Yale School of Medicine. I needed to get referred to doctors who could care for a patient like me, and so I set up the appointment. This was one of the first times I had been proactive in trying to set up appointments with doctors, and I did so because I had been spending so much time pouring over my medical records and thinking about everything Dr. Koufos did for me.

I went through the same tests as I did in Akron in 2006, and in the meetings with the doctor and nutritionist, I made jokes about the things I wasn't doing that I knew I should have been, and they asked me, like Pam had asked me ten years ago, why I was even there if I didn't care about my health going forward.

At one point, Dr. Nina Kadan-Lottick asked me if I saw the doctor who treated me when I went to the late-effect clinic in 2006.

"He died in 1998," I said, and added that he was young and that he was amazing and that I was heartbroken by his death.

"Would you have gone back if he were still alive?" she asked.

It was the first time I had ever thought about that, thought about how his death impacted me, not emotionally, because I have been thinking about that since the day he died, but medically, physically. Would I have continued seeing Dr. Koufos in Akron if he were still alive? Absolutely! I wanted him to see me be successful. I wanted him to know that he had done something special in keeping me alive. I wanted him to be proud of me. And if I had gotten the medical attention I needed at the time, then that would have been a bonus. But I let it go because he wasn't there.

It dawned on me, though, after Dr. Kadan-Lottick left the room and I sat on the exam table, staring at the wall in somewhat of a stupor, that Dr. Koufos would have been, would be, most proud of me not because of any book I write or the stories I tell about him—he did not like being the center of attention—but by my staying alive, by my not wasting the amazing work he did so long ago.

I've gotten lucky so far. In twenty-six years, the worst that has happened to me is the nineteen harmless skin cancers that have been cut off my head. But I need to acknowledge that that won't always be the case, and that's all right because that's life. The thing I need to do is guard my life as fiercely as Dr. Koufos guarded it while he was alive.

CHAPTER 22

The Search for Todd and Tim

W e were in a Chick-fil-A when my phone started ringing. The phone number was from Bluffton, South Carolina, and I wondered who could possibly be calling me from there. I initially thought it was a telemarketer, and I was going to let it go to voicemail, but then I decided to answer it, something I rarely do.

"This is Matt," I said.

"Matt, this is Bill Seitz."

It took me a second before I realized who had called me. It was Todd's dad.

About a month earlier, I had mailed a copy of "The Ghosts I Run With" and a letter explaining the book I was working on to an address I found online that most likely belonged to Todd's parents. I did the same with an address I found for Tim's parents. Like I had with Janet, Melissa and Dr. Koufos, I wanted to know more about Tim and Todd. I needed them to be more fully developed in my mind when I thought about them.

It took me a while before I was able to nail down names and addresses to send my essay to, in regard to Todd and Tim. I made several trips to the clinic to look at my medical records in the spring of 2016. I made one trip for the sole purpose of asking Pam about Todd and Tim. I had come up with nothing in my initial forays online as I searched for who they were and who their parents were, something that was disappointing but not unexpected. Todd, Tim, and even Melissa existed in a world before Google and the Internet. They died before newspapers put obituaries online, before people posted things on Facebook asking their friends to share a photo of this sick kid and to think about them. When I did Google searches for Tim and included

Akron Children's Hospital, the only thing that came up was the *Good Morning America* video segment that I uploaded to YouTube after having it digitized, and an Associated Press article that ran in newspapers around the country about *Road to Remission*, most notably in the *Los Angeles Times*. As for Todd, well, there is nothing.

At the very least, I needed their parents' names because that could start me down the right path. But it's been more than twenty years since Todd and Tim passed away, and Pam couldn't find any information that would help. She didn't remember either of Todd's or Tim's parents' names. She said she thought that they both moved away. She said she saw Tim's parents at his calling hours, and then they seemed to drop off the face of the earth. She said Todd's parents took his ashes and started spreading them on the greatest golf courses in the United States, including Augusta, before they moved to Florida. She thought.

Pam told me what she thought Todd's mom's name was, and I wrote it down in the hope it might knock something loose in Google's search engine. It didn't. I asked Pam if she knew when Tim died. I thought if I had something close to a date, I might be able to find his obituary in an archived copy of the *Akron Beacon Journal*, but she couldn't come up with that.

Ultimately, I found the information in the most logical place possible, in the *Akron Beacon Journal* online archives, something I found out far later than I should have. I had to pay for them, which is one reason why my Google searches did not bring them to me. But those obituaries gave me Todd's and Tim's parents' names. I did a few public records searches and landed on the addresses I mailed "The Ghosts I Run With" to.

I didn't hear anything for the longest time and started to think the addresses were wrong. It had been so easy to get in touch with the families of my other ghosts. In fact, they had contacted me. But I was having a hard time getting in touch with anyone from Todd's or Tim's family. In many ways, they had simply up and disappeared according to everyone I talked with at the hospital. By the time Bill called, I was ready to give up on ever finding anything out about Todd and Tim.

"We've been traveling for a while and just got home and gotten your package," Bill said. "It's very exciting what you're doing with your life."

By now, I had moved to a table in a corner of Chick-fil-A..

"How did you find our address?" Bill asked, but not in a way that made me think he was annoyed that I found their address.

"I used to be a reporter," I said. "I can usually find just about anything."

"I'll bet you can," he said and laughed.

His voice. There was something in his voice that made me think I was hearing an echo of Todd.

Bill and I made small talk. He asked how my family ended up in Sandy Hook, Connecticut, which he knew from the return address on the envelope I mailed him. I told Bill that we had just moved recently. When he called me, we had been gone from Ohio for less than two months. He asked if I had kids, and I told him about Emery and Lily.

I told Bill that I definitely wanted to talk with him more, but that at that moment, I had nothing to take notes with. I told him I had memories of Todd, and I wanted to know if they were accurate portrayals of his son.

"It's been just about twenty-four years," Bill said, and I could tell, even though we were a thousand miles away, that he was starting to choke up.

A month later, I still hadn't called Bill back. In so many ways, I feel like I am intruding on these people's lives, like I am forcing them to pull off a scab and expose a wound that has been trying to heal for more than two decades. Even though I tell myself it's so other people can know how wonderful their loved ones are, and I know that they appreciate the opportunity to talk to someone about the person they lost, it's still hard. I tell myself, I'll call tomorrow, and when tomorrow comes, I say, I'll call tomorrow. It's not laziness and it's not even procrastination. I don't know what it is.

And then I got a letter. It was late October. It was from Tim's dad, Jack Snyder. The letter was about a page long. It described Tim's illness, how it started and how it ended.

"Tim's cancer started with back pain," Jack wrote. "We thought it might be growing pains because he was already over six feet. We took him to Akron Children's Hospital, where they discovered that he had a tumor on his kidney. The tumor ruptured and he was considered Stage 4; it took several months to find what type of tumor it was."

It was, ultimately, an incredibly rare type of tumor, Jack said, one they had to treat like Ewing sarcoma. The first tumor was removed, but immediately, doctors realized there was a second tumor they had missed. He had to have another surgery.

All of this happened before I ever met Tim. This is, incredibly, not the story of how he ultimately died. This is how he came to be the type of kid who would say, "I wish I would've had a game to play so I would've known what to expect."

In the same video that I go to when I want to hear Todd's voice, I can hear Tim's. I can see Tim, and he is healthy and vibrant. He was two years younger than me, and we were both in the hospital at the same time. In the video, we are sitting beside each other as we play the game for the cameras. We both have plenty of hair, but we are also both wearing hats. In this video, we have both finished the game. We have both survived.

"Tim had roughly four and a half good years before the cancer reappeared," Jack wrote.

Jack also included a photo of Tim, his senior picture. He's wearing a jacket and tie. His hair is combed perfectly. He's got a slightly open mouth. He looks like he is about to tackle life in the same way he tackled being a sick teenager, and that was by doing something that landed him on national television.

Pam said that Tim's death was one of the hardest for so many at Akron Children's Hospital because he had been doing so well. In the *Good Morning America* segment, taped on March 2, 1993, he was strong and vibrant. He had a whole life in front of him, until he didn't.

After I received Jack's letter, I decided it was time to make calls. I called Bill Seitz first and left a message. Bill called back a couple days later. It turns out, I had called him in the aftermath of Hurricane Matthew, and he and his wife lived in Hilton Head, South Carolina, which was hit hard by the storm. He laughed when I mentioned my realization of what I had done, and he said they rode the storm out. I thought of Todd on that horse as he was falling, just laughing and having the time of his life. Of course Todd's parents would not run from a hurricane. They would experience it, just like Todd fully experienced everything he encountered.

Bill immediately started talking about the horseback riding incident at Camp CHOPS. I didn't even have to bring it up. He said Todd couldn't stop talking about it when he got home from camp that weekend.

"He thought it was funnier than heck," Bill said.

"All these people were sitting there in awe of me," Todd told his parents.

I told Bill I remembered Todd just laughing manically as he sat on the ground, and asked him if he thought that was something Todd would have done.

"Oh, absolutely," Bill said. "He was an upbeat man."

I never got more than just the letter from Jack Snyder. I left him voicemail messages and sent him emails and didn't hear back. I didn't press hard because I didn't know what kind of anguish I may have been causing him. I thought about what Pam told me, that Tim's death was the hardest out of all of the ones she had seen. He had been healthy for more than four years. When I was four years out, I was suffering through the summer of 1995, working in a factory I didn't want to be at, living in a house that contained just one of my parents, drinking far too much alcohol for someone who wasn't twenty-one years old yet and whose liver had already been through so much. And yet, I knew that I was alive and figured that I would always be so, at least for a while, and that it wouldn't end because of the disease I had just fought off.

But it did come back for Tim, and he fought and fought and fought and still lost. He was twenty years old when he died. He was thirteen when he was diagnosed. I try to imagine the anguish his parents went through, first when his cancer was found and then when it was seemingly defeated, how euphoric they must have been to see their son on national television, talking about being on the swim team and about inventing a game that could help thousands of kids and families. What gratitude they must have felt as they sent him off to college. And how far did they crash when the disease returned? Tim had faith in God. His father told me so in the letter he wrote me. I imagine his parents had the same faith. But those must have been incredibly dark days, darker than I can even imagine.

And here I am, asking them to relive them.

Todd was born in October 3, 1975, just about a month and a half before me, and Bill said it was obvious from the start that he had a personality. He was a carefree kid who wanted to experience everything life had to offer. That didn't change when he found out he had cancer. It happened after he was playing peewee football as an eight-year-old and his knee became swollen. They went to the doctor and found that he had osteogenic sarcoma. His leg would have to be amputated above the knee.

After the surgery, Todd started swimming. Then he got involved in skiing with a club called the Three Trackers, a group of amputees who skied. When he was fourteen, Todd was featured on ESPN's *Scholastic Sports* show because he won three silver medals and a bronze medal at the National Championships for Disabled Skiers. He told a reporter then that being on national television was no big deal.

He was befriended by Edward DeBartolo Jr., a Youngstown native who owned, at the time, the San Francisco 49ers. That happened after Todd wrote a letter to quarterback Joe Montana and never got a reply. Someone at Akron Children's knew someone who knew someone who knew DeBartolo, and the next thing Todd and his family knew they were flying out to San Francisco for football games.

"He has done more for me to help me fight to stay alive then I ever expected him to," Todd wrote about DeBartolo in a paper for school on friendship.

After a while, he picked up golf and decided it was better than skiing because he was never cold. He became the manager of the football team at Ellet High School in Akron. He loved going to school and hated the fact that he missed so much. From the time he had his leg amputated to the time I met him, he had had so many other surgeries to remove the tumors that kept coming back. He had part of his shoulder removed, as well as some ribs and one lung. He was almost always bald.

"He liked being around the kids, mainly," Bill said.

And kids, as well as teachers, loved being around Todd. Regina Brett, a columnist for the *Akron Beacon Journal*, wrote about Todd a handful of times, including after he died. While I may have read one or two of these pieces back when they were originally written, I didn't remember them and only happened upon them when I paid for access to the *Beacon Journal* archives.

"He was always willing to talk to other children who were diagnosed. He'd take off his shirt and show them how to get chemotherapy," Pam said to Brett for that story.

Todd died on a Sunday. Brett's column ran three days later.

"On Monday," she wrote, "the school library was full of crying students."

The students created a memorial scholarship fund in his name.

Bill has a lasting image of his son, and it comes from less than a week before Todd died. He said they were waiting to see a doctor at the hospital, when Todd looked over at another sick boy.

"Hey Dad," Todd said, "I'm sure glad I don't have what that kid over there has. He looks bad. He's not going to make it."

As I talked with Bill, I found myself wanting to tell him about what I went through. I told him about Dr. Koufos and what Camp CHOPS meant to me. I told him that even though it had been been twenty-five years, I couldn't stop thinking about the days when I was sick. I only knew Todd from the handful of times the support group met, from that one year at Camp CHOPS when he fell off the horse, and the recording of the video segment for *Road to Remission*.

There is one thing I would love to know about Tim.

How did he come up with the idea for *Road to Remission?* The video segment and the spot on *Good Morning America* all give a stock answer, that he thought, as he was being treated for his first tumor, that there should be a board game that would help him understand what he was going through. I certainly believe that. But how did he get to that place? How did he get through the surgeries, the chemotherapy, and the nurses waking him up in the middle of the night to get to a place of thinking about other kids, those who would come after him with the same horrific issues? I wish I could say that I had that kind of empathy then, that I thought about people other than myself. But I didn't. I withdrew. In the sixty-seven days I stayed at Akron Children's, plus all the other days I stayed there after the initial residency, I didn't once walk down to the recreation room on the fourth floor, where many of the kids receiving chemotherapy went to hang out together. Not once. In my days as a patient at Akron Children's, I didn't once interact with another kid, and I certainly don't think I thought about any others, except for maybe that baby that always seemed to be alone in a crib in the room next to 462.

It goes to show how special of a person Tim was, which I think also gets back to why his death was just so damn hard for so many people to take.

Bill told me about a Christmas party that was held at St. Bernard's Church in downtown Akron. The church was across the street from the hospital, and the Hematology and Oncology Department held the party for its patients. There was a girl who was a couple years older than Todd, who, at the time, would have been sixteen, and she asked him to take her to the prom that following May. Todd leaped at the opportunity in the way a boy with only one leg could. A month after that prom, he would fall off a horse. Five months after the prom he would die.

As Bill told this story, I was flooded with memories of that party because I was there too, although I hadn't thought about it in a very long time. I remember walking into the church with Mom. It was on a day when I had already received treatment in the clinic. The room we were in seems like it was big but maybe not. We sat at a table and had some food and cake. We talked with each other, sick kids commiserating about our treatments and parents leaning on each other for support. Then Santa Claus showed up with presents for all of us kids. I don't know what my present was. But I do know that when I looked Santa Claus in the eyes, they were a deep, soft brown, eyes that I had looked into so many times, and the hands that reached into the red bag were red and chaffed, and his "Ho, Ho, Ho" was more of a "Ho, Ho," chuckle.

Bill sent me a packet in the mail about two months after we talked on the phone. He included in the packet several things that Todd had written, as well as stories that were written about him: the dedication page to his high school yearbook the year he died, several *Akron Beacon Journal* stories, and more.

His writing was similar to my own, in the sense that cancer came up in just about every subject he wrote about. He brought it up in his essay on friendship. "There have been many people who touched my life in these 16 painful years that I have lived," he wrote.

He brought it up when he wrote about himself, obviously. "Courage is another trait that I feel I have," he wrote. "I think of myself as being courageous because I have been battling for my life since I was eight. I have been battling the traumatic disease, Cancer. I feel that it takes a lot of courage to battle for your life like I have. It has been an up hill battle since the beginning, and I'm not about to give up."

He even brought cancer up when he wrote a piece about the ocean titled "New Frontiers."

"In the past year," he wrote, "we have made fascinating discoveries. I know of one for sure that definitely makes me feel that it is worth while to explore the sea, that is many scientists believe that the shark holds the secret to a possible cure for cancer. They believe this to be true because it is a well known fact that sharks live on red meat, and yet no shark has ever developed cancer as far as we know."

Bill also sent me a photocopy of a handwritten letter from a Mrs. Martin. It was dated November 10, 1993, almost a full year after Todd died. Mrs. Martin identifies herself in the letter as the mom of Sharon, from Camp CHOPS.

"Sharon was very upset about Todd's death," Mrs. Martin wrote.

She included in the letter a photograph.

"Sharon has a copy of this picture in her dorm room at college," she wrote. "This is a close knit group of kids as you can see they were all having a great time."

Bill photocopied the photo with the letter. It's from Camp CHOPS, 1992. The year Todd fell off the horse. All six of us are in the photo: I'm on the far left, wearing my Cubs T-shirt and a Cubs hat. Kim is next to me, and

Ben is next to her. Sharon is in the middle, with Todd, wearing a T-shirt that says "I got a hole in one at Augusta," beside her and Melissa beside him. I had never seen that photo before. It was taken the same day we stood in the basket of the hot air balloon because we're all wearing the same clothes. Unlike the photo in the balloon, where we all stood, staring stone-faced into the camera, in this photo, we all have huge smiles on our faces. Our arms are draped around each other and we are frozen in time, completely happy to have found each other.

CHAPTER 23

Melissa's Faith

Louise showed me some pages from Melissa's diary when I visited her one day. She told me she had read it all after Melissa passed away. So much of it was incredibly personal, and she felt she could never share it all. While I would have liked to have read it, to understand Melissa at a level I could never have imagined, I also knew that it wasn't my right to understand her like that, that I didn't need that level of intimacy. But Louise shared a few pages with me, pages she thought I would find interesting, including her first entry after the cancer had come back. This was nine months after the diagnosis, a long stretch of time when Melissa refused to put into writing everything that she was fighting against, all of the emotions that were generated by that news, her anger at her parents, her not talking to her Dad for three months, her yelling and screaming at Louise. I've tried to imagine Dr. Koufos telling Melissa the news that she had relapsed, and I've tried imagining what her reaction was. How does one deal with that knowledge? It must have been similar to Dr. Koufos receiving his own diagnosis.

"Well, a lot has happened to me since I last made an entry," she wrote.

She detailed how her first year of college went, recorded her grade point averages. "I missed taking my spring quarter finals," she wrote. "The reason I missed taking my finals was because I was in the hospital having surgery—my cancer had returned!!"

She punctuated it with two exclamation points, I think, to note shock more than excitement. Although, in some ways, the sentence reads like something a person might write when they get a surprise visit from a loved one. Her reference to "my cancer" strikes me as incredibly true. It was her visitor, much like Janet's stranger within, a visitor who had left but not before writing a note saying maybe he would return, maybe he wouldn't. *You'll know I when I come back,* the note would have said. It strikes me now, as I write this, as very New Testament, something Jesus told the disciples as he ascended up to heaven after coming back from the dead. But that couldn't have been her intention. The only good thing that can result in cancer coming back is the knowledge that it has come back. Those of us who were diagnosed as teenagers were old enough to understand the doctors when they talked about how initial remission didn't mean we were cured, when they talked about relapses and what would happen if for some reason the cancer did in fact return. Because we could understand this talk, we lived uneasily even when we were cancer-free. We lived knowing that life could end at any moment. We learned to expect the unexpected, to never get too comfortable or to get too close, because the life we built after cancer could all come crumbling down, and it could start with a stomachache or a back pain or a headache or exhaustion.

I continue to live my life like this. I wonder, when a pain shows up in my shoulder or my knee or somewhere else in my body, if it's the beginning of the end. When I can't shake a cough, I'm reminded of those days in November and December of 1990. One of the reasons I started running in 2013 was because I was convinced I was going to drop dead before my fiftieth birthday for an odd combination of reasons, including my medical history and the weight I had gained. I'm in much better shape now. I feel healthier, but I also know that doesn't always make a difference.

Melissa says she spent three months in the hospital, and I think about that photo of us in front of the dining hall at Camp CHOPS. How soon after leaving camp did she end up in the hospital? And even worse, how did I never know this? Or did I know this and simply push it out of my brain because it was information that was just too difficult to process, too horrible to retain.

"This time however was much different than the first!" Melissa wrote. "The first time I got sick, I knew I was going to get better, but I never had that 'feeling' this time. Needless to say, I was right to feel this way.

"I'm going to die."

Melissa had another entry in which she wrote a cramped, five-page note that debated with herself as to when the right time to die would be. When I read these pages, I think about the time Melissa rode home from a chemotherapy treatment and asked her dad when she was going to die. In her diary, Melissa said she was having a conflict between her flesh and her spirit. She said her flesh was ready to die but her spirit was not. She wanted to be in perfect harmony before she left, and to obtain that perfect harmony, she laid out a four-step plan.

"1. TRAVEL—Go to places that I've always wanted to go to, and that I truly feel are necessary to go to.

"2. MEET PEOPLE—I feel that there are people that have the help & knowledge that I need for the bond in these places I feel drawn to.

"3. REMEMBER—People I'll meet will tell me things that are crucial to helping me bond and in me helping others bond, like Laura Jo's quote 'Everyone goes through a tragedy in their life, I'm just going through mine early.'

"4. STOP TREATMENTS—When I feel that the first three things have been completed as much as possible and only then . . . Start to get myself ready and to teach people what I have learned and show them by taking this action I am doing what my purpose is. But I must realize two things . . . 1. These things have NO time limits and this combines with 2. God is the One that decides if any of these things are true or necessary, cause according to this account & this book my spirit & God TOGETHER chose my PATH and He will 'remind me' if I clearly ask if these decisions are what we agreed upon."

While Melissa was writing this, while she was contemplating the end of her life, I was finishing up high school and getting ready to start what I thought was a new life. I read this and wonder, though, what I would have done had I relapsed. What if I had to come to the conclusion that I was going to die, and it was going to happen soon. Would I have done this soul searching? Would I have developed a plan, a plan that would have allowed me to come to terms with death, to try and control death, to make death come to me when I was ready? Would I have wanted to prepare my parents for my death? Or would I have just said fuck it, like I pretty much did while I was in the hospital, when I felt like I was fine with dying simply because I wanted there to be an ending to the ordeal?

For so long, I thought Melissa and I were clones, and that's why her death was always so hard for me. But I know now we were polar opposites.

She was friends with so many people, and she worked hard to maintain friendships, whether they were kids from her high school or teens she met at the hospital. One of her friends was Laura Jo. I knew Laura Jo but only in the most minor sense. We were sick at the same time. We both attended the same support group and worked on *Road to Remission*. But I never really talked with her. I never got to know her the way it seems Melissa did. In fact, I never really got to know anyone there the way it seems Melissa got to know Laura Jo. I knew Melissa better than any other patient, but as I look back, I see that I didn't know her well either. We hung out over the course of a couple weekends and one Saturday night in our lives. We talked on the phone a handful of times. But I didn't know her.

I see this, twenty-six years later, as the story of my life. I have surrounded myself with people I call friends but who I vaguely know. I've never had the type of friend who knew all my darkest secrets, who I confided in. I would say, right now, my wife is my best friend, but I also know I am a horrible friend. I won't say anything unless prompted to. I live inside my head and often find it difficult to get out. Aside from my wife, my second-best friend is Mike, a former roommate in college. He lives in Tennessee, and we try to go to a major professional golf tournament together every couple years. I talk to Mike a couple times a year, maybe. Other than that, we chat online or exchange text messages, maybe once a month. That is whom I consider my second best friend in the world. What does that say about me?

Melissa, though, she clearly knew Laura Jo. She wrote an essay about Laura Jo titled "My Hero" for one of her English classes at Ohio University. While I frequently find myself thinking about Laura Jo (especially when I watch the *Good Morning America* clip on *Road to Remission*, or when I am actually looking at the game itself), the only thing I really know about her comes from this paper Melissa wrote in college, which Louise gave to me.

Laura Jo had Ewing sarcoma, a type of bone cancer often diagnosed in teenagers. Had I actually talked to Laura Jo once or twice, had I made the effort to get out of my head and get to know more people, I would have found that Laura Jo and I had a lot in common, starting with the fact that we both wanted to be writers.

"She wrote poems and stories with brilliance and imagery that exceeded her years," Melissa wrote in her paper. "This talent, I know, helped her handle her cancer better."

Melissa mentions Laura Jo's quote in this paper as she does in her diary, and then talks about how Laura Jo's one wish was to be published.

Ultimately, the Starlight Foundation, a group that grants wishes to terminally ill children, connected Laura Jo with Erma Bombeck, who ultimately turned her nationally syndicated column over to the young cancer patient.

I found that column online. I wonder, given how much I liked to write and how much I read the local newspaper, I never realized that Laura Jo had also wanted to be a writer, indeed that she even knew who Erma Bombeck was. How did I not know she had been a part of one of Bombeck's columns until a quarter-century later, after I read an essay Melissa wrote for a college English class?

"Laura Jo Mounsey wants my job," Bombeck begins the column. "She is 15. When I was 15, I wanted my job, so I relate to her."

Then Bombeck outlines Laura Jo's situation, and turns the column over to her.

"I feel that I may cease to live not very much longer from now," Laura Jo wrote. "I also feel that before I die, I would like to feel success, to taste fame, to touch a part of the world, leave my mark and never be forgotten there."

This is a feeling I have lived my entire life with, one that has driven me, has oftentimes caused me to focus more on work than on more important things like family, love, and friendship. Like Laura Jo, I want people to know my name. I want them to look at my body of work and feel like they're looking at greatness. I want people one hundred years from now to know my name, and this started once I became a survivor of childhood cancer. As kids like Laura Jo and Melissa started dying, I felt I had to justify my own survival. Surely, making sure everyone remembered Matt Tullis would have sufficed. But now, I want something different. I want people to know Melissa's name and Laura Jo's name and the names of Janet, Alex, Todd, Tim, and so many more. I want the world to know these people in a way I didn't two decades ago.

There's another way in which Melissa and I are strikingly different. In her diary, she shows a faith that God will guide her to the right decision when it comes to stopping treatments. I don't remember talking about faith and God much around Melissa at Camp CHOPS or even on the phone, but that doesn't mean we didn't. When I was sick, I was a regular churchgoer. I grew up in the Nazarene Church, going to Sunday school and church every Sunday morning, often heading back to church for Sunday evening services, and then going in on Wednesday nights. By the time I became sick, I was active in my church's youth group. I believed wholeheartedly, at the time, that the reason

I survived was because God wanted me to survive, because he had plans for my life going forward. This belief was fortified by the people at my church talking to me about the miraculous nature of my survival.

Once, I was playing basketball at a local YMCA. One of the guys playing basketball knew about my survival because his kids went to the same school as my brothers and me. He was also a truck driver, and so he knew my dad. At one point, in between games, we were standing under a basket and he looked at me and said, "You know God has great plans for you." In so many ways, it played into my desire to have people know my name, to know who Matt Tullis was.

I didn't really know what to say in that gymnasium. What should you say to that? Thank you? I know? I've got this? I don't remember anything else about that moment. The only thing that sticks with me from that day is that one line.

Given my nature, this idea that God had special plans for me, that he had singled me out, had seen me and decided I was special, played right into the mindset of a young man who really did want to be special. So I ran with that idea of the miraculous teenager all the way through high school until I reached college. I'm not sure why, but once I got to college, I didn't want to be different anymore. I wanted to fit in. I think just about all college students go through that process. And as I was busy trying to fit in, trying not to be singled out by God, I started realizing all of these kids I knew were dead or dying. Melissa's death was the one that pushed me into the realm of questioning whether I believed in God or not, and Dr. Koufos's death sent me spiraling over the edge. I stopped believing in God precisely because of this idea that I might be worth saving, but they weren't.

Melissa's dad, Jim, a retired military man, tears up when he talks about his daughter, specifically about her faith. He told me about her faith and his faith that God was only doing what was in his plan, and his plan was always good.

"My pastor told me God doesn't make mistakes," Jim said, wiping his eyes with a tissue, and Melissa believed that wholeheartedly.

I think about how Melissa faced adversity after adversity and never lost the belief that what was happening was supposed to be happening. Her faith sustained her even after being told her cancer had come back, even after she had intuited that she was going to die. And she wasn't the only one. Tim's father wrote in a letter to me that his son "became a born again Christian," and that his faith gave him strength and optimism. Janet wrote about knowing God's peace and that only he could silence the cancer that had invaded her body. Todd's dad told me "that God works in mysterious ways, and we just need to accept the outcome. Our family is very close, and we believe that is because of Todd and his courage and faith."

They all had faith. They believed, even as they were weakened by disease, as they were broken down. Their faith was the thing that made them strong enough to face the end, and I'm happy they had that. This has created a paradox in my own mind, though, because as they died, their faith was strengthened. But when they died, my faith was destroyed.

I still don't believe in God, but the faith of my ghosts helps smooth the sharp edges I've developed when it comes to a higher power. It makes me wonder if someday I will come back around. I am constantly thinking about this topic and what it means for my life, for all of our lives. But I don't believe now. That doesn't mean God didn't exist to Melissa and the others, and that is an important thing for me to consider, to understand. I hesitate to even bring up the idea of faith (and my lack of it) given how strong it seems Melissa's faith was. But it wouldn't be faithful to my story and Melissa's to ignore it. Indeed, it's been my lack of faith that has driven me to the point I'm at primarily because I've voided the idea that there were preordained plans for me. I was devastated when I finally came to the conclusion that God didn't have plans for me, that there was no explanation as to why I was still walking on this planet and Melissa and Laura Jo and Tim and Todd and all of those other kids and Dr. Koufos and Janet were not.

When I came to that conclusion, I was lost. I was a soul on this planet with nowhere to go, with nothing to do but deal with the fact that there was no order to the chaos. I was left to make my own order, to create my own understanding. That knowledge led me to where I am at now, to my need for understanding exactly what I went through and to tell the stories of the people who meant so much to me, people I never actually told they meant so much to me, people whose families I hope can take solace in knowing that someone they've never heard of is still carrying the memories of their loved ones around in his heart and mind on a daily basis.

Louise gave me a bunch of the photos of Melissa that she showed me the first time I met her. In some of them Melissa is completely healthy. There is one portrait that appears to have been taken before she was ever sick, where her hair falls below her shoulders and she's wearing a suit coat. There's another where she is holding flowers and is obviously getting ready to go out for the night. Her hair in that photo is much shorter but not because she is sick. Rather, it's just a different cut.

There are also a couple of photos from Camp CHOPS, including the one of us all standing in the gravel driveway that led to the mess hall. I like these photos the most because they show the Melissa I see when I think of her. Short hair. Great, beaming smile. I imagine her getting ready to laugh or start talking about something in this incredibly loud voice, a voice that carried, a voice that demanded you pay attention to what it had to say.

There is, in this collection of photos, one that includes me that I had never seen before. This photo sums up my life and what I know of Melissa more than anything else. In the photo, Melissa is in the foreground. She is sitting under a tent at Camp CHOPS. It is a Sunday afternoon, during the final ceremonies, where counselors get up and give silly awards to all the campers. Melissa is staring straight into the camera. Her hair is fuzzy and she looks far skinnier than in other Camp CHOPS photos, which means it was taken in 1994, just about a year after she found out her cancer had returned and six months before she died. For a long time, I thought that the last time I saw Melissa was at Camp CHOPS in 1993, just before she found out her cancer came back. I had no memory of seeing her in 1994 and have lived thinking that she never came back. I found out only recently when Sharon, who I reconnected with on Facebook, showed me a photo of her and Melissa from camp that year. In that photo, Melissa looks a lot like she does in the photo I'm in, a photo I long thought was taken just as I was about to become a senior in high school and not a freshman in college.

In the photo from the Sunday ceremony, Melissa is smiling as little kids shove lollipops into their mouths just behind her. The closing ceremonies of camp were always one of the best times of the weekend because we got to tell funny stories about the campers as their parents all stood in the background and watched their sick children laugh and pretend to be normal.

I stand in the background, on the far left side of this photo. I look strong, like someone who was never sick at all. When the photo was taken, I was just about a week away from graduating from high school. Whoever was taking this photo was not trying to squeeze me into the frame. It just happened. I'm photobombing before photobombing was a thing. I'm frozen there, standing in a red shirt and hat with sunglasses on. I'm not inside the tent. I'm outside, just looking in. I'm a bystander, silent, off to the side. For so long, I've tried to claim some part of Melissa's life as my own, but it's really only ever been this tenuous grasp, a guy standing off in the background, quite by accident. I have no claim to her at all, or any of the others, other than this knowledge that we encountered each other at a time when I was still as vulnerable as I think I have ever been, and Melissa and the others left a lasting impression on me. In some ways, the photo exhibits the opposite of that. She is there in the foreground, and I am there in the background. Which maybe is perfect, a way to show the relationship we had together, never perfectly together, but always there, just off to the left. I'm there and she is there and we will be there forever.

CHAPTER 24

Back to Clinic

I went back to the clinic on a day in March 2016. Pam had requested my medical records so I could look at them, and they had come in and were sitting on her desk. When I was a patient, Pam was the woman who administered medicine to patients. Now she's running a part of the hematology and oncology clinic that deals with long-term side effects of chemotherapy and radiation on childhood cancer patients. It had been ten years since I had gone back for a comprehensive checkup that looked at the ways the treatments that had saved my life were taking a toll on my body now, ten years since Pam told me I needed to change my lifestyle if I wanted to have the chance at a long life.

But this visit was to look at my records. I had done the same thing in 2004, when I was in graduate school. Back then, I had gone through the official channels at the hospital and sat in a tiny room in the Medical Records office looking through the detailed notes of my life as a childhood cancer patient. I had marked about two hundred pages and paid more than $50 for copies to be made. Thanks to the changes in technology since that first visit with my records, I could take pictures of any of the pages I wanted with my phone. And because I was working in Pam's office, I could ask her questions whenever one popped up.

I walked into the clinic at about 10 a.m. Pam was working with patients, so I sat in the waiting room for about thirty minutes. I had been in this clinic before, the new clinic, which by now wasn't so new but that would always be new in my mind because it wasn't the clinic I visited as a patient. I had never sat in this waiting room for the amount of time I did on that morning, though, and I was fine with that. I watched a girl of Indian descent, perhaps about ten years old, sit and watch the flat-screen television, which was on the Disney Junior channel. She had a fleece hat pulled over her bald head, and she occasionally blew a plastic whistle that she twirled in her hands. Her mom had been there when I walked in but was gone now. She returned after about fifteen minutes with coffee, but for a while, I watched the girl and tried to remember what it was like to be a patient, sitting, waiting, knowing that I was there to get more drugs pumped into my body.

As I watched that girl, I realized that the day was pretty close to the twenty-fifth anniversary of when I actually left the hospital as an in-patient and started visiting the clinic on a regular basis. I have those dates saved on my phone for reasons I can't even come close to explaining, so I pulled it out and checked. Sure enough, I was released from Akron Children's Hospital on March 13, 1991. My first visit to clinic as an outpatient happened two days later. It was now March 18, 2016. I was three days past the twenty-fifth anniversary of my first visit to clinic. Because I am a journalist, and journalists love anniversaries that end in a zero or a five, especially those like twenty-five, I felt my breath escape my lungs and struggled to regain it. I pictured myself, sitting in the hallway waiting room down on the second floor where the clinic used to be, those white, barren walls, the hard plastic chairs, the excruciating wait. As I thought about those things, I wanted nothing more than to go over and hug that little girl, to tell her it would be all right, that she would be all right. I wanted to push the fears out of her that she no doubt felt. But I couldn't, for so many reasons, but the primary one being that I didn't know that it would be all right for her.

I made several trips to Akron from March through May of 2016 to look at those records. On my last trip, I didn't really need to look at the records, other than to confirm a date or two. Mainly, I wanted to talk with Pam and ask her a couple questions related to my records. I hoped she would be able to explain some of the more confusing things in them. I also hoped she would be able to decipher nurse signatures. I had long ago figured out which nursing flow charts had been filled out by Janet because her signature was large and flowing and included her hyphenated last name of Creech-Forrer. But there were other nurses whose names I couldn't figure out, and I really wanted to know what days Theresa took care of me versus Joan or John or Beth. Additionally, I wanted to get copies of the flow charts from the days Janet took care of me, if for no other reason than I wanted to be able to look at her loopy cursive writing anytime I found myself thinking of her. I wanted to be able to see tangible proof that our lives had intersected.

At one point, we started talking about Todd and Tim and then she got very quiet. She has been a nurse who cared for kids with cancer for so long and has seen far too many of those kids die. A couple years before this visit, Pam told me that she was going to leave pediatric hematology and oncology and become a nurse in a podiatrist's office because nobody ever died of foot or ankle problems. But she didn't. She was still here. On this visit to the clinic, after we moved on from Todd and Tim, she told me the reason she kept doing what she was doing was because of me, because of the hope I gave her that even the sickest kids could survive.

She said that every week while I was in the hospital Dr. Koufos gave a report on his patients on the fourth floor. This included reports on me from January through March of 1991. And every week, it seemed to get worse, Pam said. She remembers thinking there was no way I would ever survive, but I kept surviving.

"We started calling you the Energizer Bunny because you kept going," she said. "There was something in your constitution that refused to give up."

And that, she said, is why she has not given up.

I was on the second volume of records when I came across pages from Wooster Community Hospital. Included in this is a Pediatric Nursing History Assessment, in which Mom filled out everything from my immunization history and previous hospitalizations to my "pets or favorite toys at home" and whether or not I was able to bathe and feed myself. These notes also included the consent form that Mom signed, allowing Dr. Spiess to do a bone marrow aspiration and biopsy, which she signed at 6:05 p.m. on January 2, 1991, just about four hours after I entered the hospital. There is a blood count, the first one taken in a hospital, that shows my white blood count was at 139.5 (a normal count would be between five and ten). That blood was drawn at 3:10 p.m., less than an hour after I was admitted to the hospital. The results were recorded at 4:38 p.m.

I had wanted to find these records for a very long time, and it turns out they were always right there, in the records I had looked at in 2004 when I was in grad school, and they were there in 1997 when I met with Dr. Koufos. I've wanted to see them because they represent the beginning, when it all started. They document the final days of precancerous Matt Tullis, of the boy I was before my illness destroyed me and my doctors and nurses saved me.

I've long been fascinated with the fact I watched *Hoosiers* while at Wooster Community Hospital. I was a small-town kid facing the biggest challenge in my life, and I was going to have to head off to the big city in order to overcome that challenge. The night I watched the movie would end up being one of only two nights I spent by myself in the hospital, the other being the one night in intensive care.

In the records, the nurse notes that I was watching a "movie video," on that first night in the hospital. I've long remembered her sitting in the room with me, watching the movie, and just being present. I remember taking comfort in the fact she was there. But this is what I didn't remember and what I wouldn't confront until this day at the clinic: "Patient cried briefly. Did not say anything to nurse." And later, at midnight: "Patient very quiet does not offer any comments. Has tears in eyes."

I read this while sitting alone in Pam's office, and tears formed in my eyes again. My breaths grew shallow, and I fought to keep from sobbing. I was thinking about the utter helplessness that I must have felt that night. I don't remember feeling that way, and I can't even begin to delve back into my fifteen-year-old brain to try to understand what was going through my mind then. What did I know about the disease I had? Did I realize my life was never going to be the same? Did I know I might die? Or was I just scared that I was spending the night in a hospital away from my family?

Once, I drove up to the hospital to look at the records from my visits to the outpatient clinic, to see if I could spot any milestones that I remembered. On this trip, though, I got there in a little bit different fashion. Instead of driving straight up to Akron after dropping my eight-year-old daughter off at school, I drove first to Apple Creek, to the house I was living in when I was diagnosed with leukemia, the house that was the starting point for every single trip to the clinic. That was about a twenty-mile drive in itself, but I wanted to recreate the journey as much as I could. I wanted to see if making that specific drive knocked anything loose in my mind.

I've been back to Apple Creek a lot since Mom and Dad sold the house after they divorced. My brother John still lives in the area, just a couple miles outside of the small village. Alyssa's grandma lived there until she moved into assisted living before passing away. In fact, her grandma lived less than a quarter-mile from the house I grew up in. As a young adult who was just starting out as a newspaper reporter, I spent a lot of summer days mowing Grandma Merkle's yard. Alyssa and I didn't have a washer and dryer, and Grandma needed her yard cut. It was a great partnership, one that almost always resulted in her buying me pizza when I was done. Invariably, when I left her house, I drove by my old house.

This was all before Alyssa and I moved to North Carolina, spent three years there and then moved back. Even then, the old house was in rough shape. It was built sometime in the 1920s. I used to know exactly when, but that's a piece of information that has long since washed out of my mind. For a long time, after it was first built, the house was owned by an old school-teacher who lived alone. There was a sunroom (which ended up being my first bedroom), and the old woman used to sit in that room and shoot squirrels as they scurried up the many trees that surrounded the house.

My parents bought the house in the summer of 1988. By then, the house was more than fifty years old. It was solid. Sturdy. It was our first house as a family, at least the first house my parents owned that didn't have wheels on it.

Add another twenty-five years to the house, though, and it's not doing so well. It's clear the owners are making repairs, most likely on their own. I pulled onto the street that ran beside the house, a small, dead-end street that leads to some homes owned by senior citizens and a small apartment build-ing. I circled around and stopped in front of the driveway. A long time ago, the people who bought the house put in a new driveway on the other side of the house. This led to a door that entered the kitchen. I was in front of what we had always used as the main driveway, which circled around to High Street. From here, I could see the yard that I used to throw tennis balls from, across the driveway and into the railroad ties that served as a retaining wall and helped create a raised flowerbed. Mom always got angry at me when I threw ball after ball after ball at that wall because I often missed high and shredded the flowers she had planted in the spring. Now, the ties had disintegrated entirely and the yard was full of huge piles of dirt. There used to be about six or seven trees in that yard as well, and now there were just three.

When I first got home and out of the hospital, once I was able to start moving around and could walk on my own, I went outside with my base-ball glove and a tennis ball. I didn't head for the railroad ties that first time, though, because it seemed too far to walk. Instead, there was a concrete re-taining wall on the other side of the steps that led to the front door. Whereas the railroad tie wall was separated from the grass by the eight-foot-wide gravel driveway, the concrete wall was surround by gravel. It was that concrete retaining wall that I threw a ball against for the first time after getting sick. It was my first pitch of my new life. Most likely I went out there wearing my

Air Jordans, which by now looked like canoes on my feet and skinny legs. I would have had on a Cubs hat. I threw the ball a couple of times and realized I was exhausted. I couldn't throw the ball hard and I could barely reach down to scoop it up when it came scooting back to me. But I had done it and I remember feeling a sense of accomplishment, like I had reclaimed something from my past. I would go on to do that quite often in the coming summer months, the first summer I didn't play baseball since I knew that I could play baseball. I would throw the ball against that concrete, and, later, the railroad ties, again and again and again.

It took a few minutes of staring at the house, but I realized the concrete wall was gone. There was a hole at the side of the house, exposing the foundation directly below the sunroom. There was a long drainpipe leading off a gutter in the same area. Whoever owned the place now was clearly dealing with issues as the house neared its hundredth birthday.

The paint was flaking off the side of the house. I wondered if it was that same coat of paint we had put on, a couple summers after I got sick. I helped scrape and paint a bit, but once people started going up on scaffolding, I bailed. I claimed I wasn't feeling good, which still gave me pretty wide latitude to do what I wanted and skip what I didn't want to do, but really I was afraid of the heights. And it was hard work. That paint would have been put on the house sometime in 1993 or 1994, which meant it was more than twenty years old.

There was also some siding missing up on the second floor. The flowerbed, another one created by railroad ties, that I had shoveled and turned one year close to my high school graduation, was overrun with bushes and flowers. The pole that had once held our basketball hoop still stood in the driveway, but with no hoop or backboard. The basement window that John used to climb out late at night to go hang with his friends was still visible. The two giant trees—and they were giant when we owned the house—still stood in the front yard, now sporting massive trunks.

Despite its issues, it was still the place that, when I think "home," I envision. I don't know if it's because it was our first actual house or if there is something more to it, something to do with the fact that it was the place we lived when I was sick. That's the place where my life came crumbling down and then was built back up, and so it will always be my original home.

I took one of the routes to Akron Children's that Mom and I took most often when I went to clinic. This was a chilly April morning, although the sun was out. I thought it was entirely possible that Mom and I had made this drive exactly twenty-five years earlier to the day (we hadn't, although we had made the trip twenty-five years and three days ago). I took the back way out of Apple Creek and then drove on back roads all the way into Orrville. From there it was state routes and the interstate. It was exactly 36.7 miles from my old driveway to the parking deck that Mom and I always parked in.

Along the way, I was struck by how many places I passed that were associated with significant memories in my life. Some of those memories came from my life before I was sick, others after. But it seemed like every couple minutes, an internal voice was saying, *That's where _____ happened.* I passed a cemetery on Carr Road and remembered how, in kindergarten, a friend and I used to pretend that cemetery was full of dinosaur bones as we rode past on the bus. I passed the dirt track speedway that my family spent nearly every Saturday night over the course of about three summers, back before I got sick. I passed a CVS pharmacy in Orrville that, when I was a younger, was actually home to the movie theater where I saw my first movies, which I vaguely recall being *The Fox and the Hound* and *E.T.*

I drove past Viking Street, where Janet used to live, and I drove past what used to be a McDonald's but is now just an empty building. It was there I had my first birthday party, or at least the first birthday party I remember. And then a short time later, I drove past the newer McDonald's, the one Mom and I used to stop at on our way home from the clinic, where I would get a cheeseburger and a pizza, back when McDonald's served pizza. That was also the McDonald's where Janet purchased the sausage biscuits that she brought to my hospital room.

A little farther up the road, I passed the Orrville Industrial Park, which is home to the factory that I worked at during that dark summer of 1995 and that my dad drove a semi out of for a good part of my childhood. About eight miles up the road from the factory was a small truck stop. Dad used to stop there all the time, and then he lived there for a short time, in an apartment above the restaurant. Past the small town of Doylestown, where Mom—retired, but still working part-time now as a nurse in a doctor's office—lives in a house trailer once again.

I started to wonder how so many landmarks could be littered along this road to Akron Children's Hospital. The memories from before I was sick are happenstance, just a result of the fact we lived close to this town and frequently drove these roads. But all of the stuff after? Was I drawn to this trail to the hospital? Were my parents? Did we keep coming back for some reason? Is there something we are trying to find?

In April 2016, Pamela Colloff of *Texas Monthly* wrote a story about the first shooting victim in the 1966 University of Texas Tower shooting. It was the first mass shooting at a school. Colloff wrote about a woman named Claire, who was eighteen years old and pregnant when she was shot. She survived. The baby and her boyfriend did not.

The Reckoning is about how that one bullet changed the trajectory of her life. It ends with a paragraph about how Claire finds herself constantly wanting to go back to the open area where she was shot, that big expanse of concrete, and lie down. She wants to find the exact spot where she collapsed, where her boyfriend lay just feet away and died, and where her unborn baby died inside of her. She wants to lie there, to feel what that hot concrete was like again in the moment that changed her life.

"It's beyond me why I would feel comforted there," Claire told Colloff. "But I want to lie down, and remember the heat, and remember Tom, and remember the baby."

By the time I got to that sentence, I was in tears, not because of what Claire had gone through in her life, but because I knew exactly how she felt. I would give anything to be able to lie in a hospital bed in room 462 at Akron Children's Hospital and look out my window, see the intersection, and watch the front door of the Ronald McDonald house. I want to hear the screaming sirens of ambulances careening into the emergency room entrance. I want to hear the wailing IV pumps, empty and in need of replenishment. While Claire wants to be in her place to remember her unborn baby and her boyfriend, I want to be in my place because that is where the old Matt died and where a new Matt was born.

That place, that room, 462 on 4-North at Akron Children's Hospital, no longer exists. The fourth floor at the hospital is now the Pediatric Intensive Care Unit, fitting, in my case, considering I spent about twenty-four hours in that unit as a patient. The window that I spent my days looking out has since been covered by an expanded hospital. There are windows there now as well, but the building doesn't remotely resemble the one I called home for sixty-seven days.

In 2004, when I went to the hospital to look at my medical records for the first time, I visited with some of my former nurses, including Theresa.

This was when all the construction was going on that was transforming the building I knew into the building it has become. Theresa asked if I would like to go into the construction area and see my old room. I said yes, absolutely, but when we got to the doors that led into what I knew as 4-North, they were locked, and by then, it was a hard hat area only, so we couldn't have gone in even if we wanted. All I would have seen would have been a skeleton of a room, which would have been fitting, because when I lived in that room, I was a skeleton of a boy.

I brushed it off as no big deal and continued visiting with the people who saved my life, but over time, I have come to regret not finding a way onto that floor, into that room. I would have been able to at least look out that window, and that is a view I would give anything to see again. As it is, I can only see it in my mind, and even then, what I see is in no way guaranteed to be what I actually saw.

When I think about that room and my window, this is what I see: I am lying in the hospital bed closest to the window. There is a chair beside the bed, and that is where Mom or Dad usually sit. On the window ledge, there are floral arrangements. One is arranged in black and gold and is in a Pittsburgh Steelers vase. There is a box of baseball cards. There is my autographed photo of Bubby Brister, the Steelers' starting quarterback, in a cheap wooden frame that Dad picked up in the hospital gift shop. There is a television up on the wall, and under that, a bulletin board that is full of the cards people sent me. Also on that bulletin board is a clock that Mom put up because the hospital room had no clock, just like a casino, and I hated not knowing what time it was, hated not knowing how many minutes of my life was flicking away in that room, but mostly hated needing help to figure out what channel to put the television on. To my left is an empty bed, one that is used by Mom or Dad, whoever is staying with me that night. There is an IV pump and maybe even a pump attached to a feeding tube, one that pushed nutrients into my malnourished body. If I turn my head, which contains only a few strands of hair that continue to cling to my scalp, to the right, I can look out the window. There's the intersection, of Locust and State streets, although I didn't know their names when I was in the hospital. It had a blinking light, red one way and yellow the other, and cars crashed in that intersection more than once during those sixty-seven days. Maybe it was the ice or the confusion of the intersection, or maybe it was the fact that the people driving the cars through the intersection were parents whose kids were in the hospital facing life threatening diseases or injuries, and they just couldn't concentrate.

Do I remember actually seeing a crash? Hearing a crash? No, but I remember Mom and Dad talking about them, like they happened when I was asleep, and I was asleep a lot. When I think about that room, I think about how much I never moved. I just lay there. I didn't interact with the room at all. It was, for all intents and purposes, my tomb. Except I didn't die.

When I came out of the hospital, I still enjoyed the same things. I maybe even enjoyed them more. I thought I would eventually get back to being normal, and I thought I did for a long time before realizing there would never be that normalcy I sought. I had seen things. I had experienced things. And they had changed me. I was different, and I had to learn to accept that.

But what I wouldn't give to be able to go back to that room, to lie in that bed, and try to submerse myself in those memories, to feel what it was like to be that kid, and to try and understand why it is I keep being pulled back to this point in time.

There's an enclosed pedestrian bridge that spans Locust Street in Akron. It connects a parking garage and medical building to the third floor entrance of Akron Children's Hospital. I crossed that bridge on January 4, 1991. I was scared, tired, still not sure what was going on. I didn't know why I was in Akron, and I didn't know what I would face in the coming days, months, and years. I couldn't comprehend all of the ways in which, in crossing that bridge, my life would change. I couldn't comprehend that I would never be the same, or that it would take me nearly a quarter-century to realize my life was never the same, and any attempts to make it so were futile.

I think about that bridge a lot. I think about crossing it to become a patient, and then that day in March 1991 when I crossed it to go home, for good, and how immediately after Mom and I crossed it, we stopped in the pharmacy that was on the medical center and parking garage side and waited for what seemed like hours but was probably only minutes for my prescriptions to be filled. Truthfully, I think about that bridge and how once I crossed it the first time, I could never uncross it, no matter how hard I tried. Indeed, in trying to uncross it, in trying to understand and unpack everything that crossing it that first time meant, it has caused me to cross that bridge—both figuratively and literally—hundreds of more times. Because when I go to Akron Children's to visit with my old nurses or to look at my medical records or to participate in an event the hospital is having, I always park in that same old parking garage and enter the same way, despite the fact the hospital has built a new parking garage and created a new, much nicer, main entrance. I can't park anywhere else because I feel I have to always enter the hospital the same way from which I initially came. I walk across that bridge and I look out to the left and see the Ronald McDonald House. I see the space where room 462 used to look out on the intersection of Locust and State. In my mind's eye, I can see it exactly as I saw it when I crossed over the first time. And when I look forward, I see the same teal and pink carpet leading straight ahead to a welcome desk that is still staffed by elderly volunteers. I see those orange elevators immediately behind the volunteers, elevators that sometime around 9:30 a.m. on January 4, 1991, took me up as I sat in a wheelchair to the fourth floor. I still take those same elevators because I don't know any other way, nor do I want to. When I am in that space, on that bridge, walking past the desk, standing in the elevator, my heart races and everything comes back in clear bursts. Instead of making me scared or confused, I feel calm, like this is the place I am meant to be.

There is a small picnic area on the west side of Akron Children's Hospital, along Locust Street. In the morning, it sits in the shadow of the hospital, with the sun coming up in the east. The medical building and the parking garage are on the other side of the street. I sat there one morning before going in to the hospital to talk to Pam, and I looked up.

Room 462 was near the corner of the hospital. There were, I think, two more rooms between mine and the edge of the building, the side that fronts on State Street. When I was in the hospital, the outer façade was a plain white, and the windows were smaller. The building was, to be frank, ugly.

That's not the case now. Akron Children's built on to this part of the hospital many years ago. It expanded outward, a beautiful red brick façade with huge windows that look in upon, I imagine, larger rooms that are more hospitable to patients and their parents.

As I looked up, I counted four floors. And then I counted three rooms over, from left to right. And I settled on a window that was, essentially, mine. I wondered who was in that room right that very second. I wondered if they were going through anything similar to what I went through. What were they battling? Were their parents there, by their side? Did they look out the window at that intersection, hoping they might see a crash? Did they care whether they lived or died? Did they have any idea how, whatever they were battling right that very second, could end up defining their life? Or if not that, did they realize that they might defeat the disease, but they might never be able to move on from it? Did they realize they might have friends who would die from similar diseases? Did they believe in God? Or fate? Should that make a difference? What were they going to do with their life if they survived and others didn't? How would they live a life that was worthy of survival?

If I could get into that room, those are the questions I would ask the kid there because those are the questions I wish I could ask my fifteen-year-old self, to make myself start thinking about these things sooner so maybe I could one day find an answer.

For a long time, I wondered why so many soldiers request to go back to combat situations. Even soldiers who have been seriously injured oftentimes will give anything to get back on the battlefield. Other former soldiers, upon leaving the military, become journalists and find ways to embed with new units of the Army or the Marines. I could never imagine why anyone would willingly go back to the places where they nearly died.

It dawned on me one morning as I was driving, yet again, to Akron Children's Hospital, that I was doing something similar. And why? Because I wanted to tell a story, sure, but there was more. Why was I constantly drawn back to the place where I very nearly died? Why was I sitting at a picnic table directly beneath the room where all of the doctors and nurses in the hematology and oncology unit thought I would die, who were all surprised that I just kept living? Why was I looking up, thinking of ways to get back into that room, into that bed?

I was going there because that is where I feel most alive. I don't know why that is the case, I just know it is so. My heart beats faster. My vision is clearer. I feel more at home. I am comfortable there, pulling into that parking garage and walking across that bridge, going up those orange elevators, hanging out in the clinic, or sitting outside and staring at a fourth-floor window, or looking across the street at the Ronald McDonald House, or looking at that intersection. I know that I could just go there and sit and watch those spaces forever and likely be content, thinking about what had happened and looking for reason in the unreasonable.

CHAPTER 25

The Marathon

I kept running after my half-marathon, and the more I ran, the more I thought about my days as a cancer patient. The more I thought about my days as a cancer patient, the more I thought about the people I knew who didn't survive. The more I thought about those people, the more I wanted to run. And so, by June of 2014, I had signed up for my first full marathon, the Akron Marathon, and I did so in partnership with the Leukemia and Lymphoma Society's Team in Training.

I chose Akron out of the many marathons I could have chosen—marathons in locations like San Diego or Alaska—for one very specific reason. The marathon ends in Canal Park, the home of the minor league baseball team the Akron RubberDucks. Runners end the marathon by coming through the outfield wall and making a beeline for where home plate would be. More important to me, though, was the fact that runners can see Akron Children's Hospital as they cross the finish line.

I trained for sixteen weeks, running with Team in Training teammates. On the weekends, I ran with a new friend named Stu. We ran about the same pace and had a lot of the same interests. He said he'd actually read some pieces I had written for SB Nation Longform, and so we spent our long training runs talking about the Browns and the Indians and the Cavs, about writing, and about those we knew who had died of cancer.

When I ran by myself during the week, I often thought of Dr. Koufos and Melissa mostly, but also Janet, Todd, and Tim. Some days, I would go out and struggle. Once, I needed to run ten miles, and it was hot and humid. I hadn't eaten properly and didn't have a water bottle with me. I slogged through mile after mile, thinking that none of the ghosts I thought about ever considered quitting. Or maybe they had considered quitting, but pushed through it, and so they pushed me through those hard runs.

There were also wonderful, breezy runs of eight or nine miles, when I would hit the road and be consumed in thought for the hour and fifteen minutes I was running, my brain darting from talk about the stork walk to *Road to Remission* to Todd falling off a horse.

By the time the marathon rolled around in September, I was in the best shape of my life. I was down to about 165 pounds and could push myself to a six-minute mile, something I had never done before. I felt strong, ready to attack the marathon.

I found Stu at the starting line and said I would run with him for a while. He was battling an Achilles injury, though, and said he wasn't sure how long he would be able to keep up with me. We started out slowly, Stu by necessity, me because I figured it was best to take it easy in my first marathon. While I wanted to finish the race in four hours and thirty minutes, I wasn't about to take off and push myself from the start.

In mile seven, Alyssa took a photo of Stu and me running by. I opened my mouth in a huge smile and threw my hands in the air as we passed by. I had never felt so good in the seventh mile of any run, and felt like I was going to conquer this race. The miles added up. We ran along the Tow Path, which runs along the now defunct Ohio Canal, a trail that, when it was included in the marathon, was typically devoid of spectators. We pushed past mile fifteen and then sixteen. The longest Stu and I had ever run together was eighteen miles, and we did it on a brutally hot and humid day in late August, but now we passed the eighteen-mile mark and we were still together. The morning had started out chilly enough that I ran about five miles with long sleeves on, but now it was getting warmer and the humidity was creeping in.

In the twentieth mile, something magical happened. I came upon a water stop, and saw a familiar face. Nancy, my social worker from Akron Children's, was handing out cups of water to runners.

"Nancy!" I yelled.

Nancy was the one who got me involved with *Road To Remission*. She was, in so many ways, the calm in the storm that was my hospital room. She was always there, checking in on me and my parents. Then she set up the support group, which was a refuge for me at the time, giving me a group of people I could talk to about things none of my other friends could relate to. I did not hold the fact that many of those friends ultimately died against Nancy, because even though I felt for a time that I was somehow wronged by knowing them for only a short amount of time, knowing them changed my life.

"That's me," she said.

I ran up and hugged her. It was quick, and, I imagine, gross for Nancy, considering I was sweaty and nasty, having run twenty miles. I never told her whom I was, assumed, instead, that she would know. I took a cup of water and then headed off. I realized a few hundred feet down the road, after I had caught up with Stu, that Nancy may not have known who I was. It had been a very long time since we had seen each other. She stopped doing social work for kids with cancer and was now working in palliative care, which I imagine is even tougher, but exactly the type of job that needs someone like Nancy in it.

I talked to Nancy about a year after the race, and asked her if she knew who I was when I hugged her. She said she eventually made the connection, but it had taken a few minutes.

That spot where I hugged Nancy marked the longest distance I had ever run before. Three weeks before the marathon, there was a training run in Akron for people who were running the race. It was a twenty-mile run that followed much of the course. I ran alone, since Stu was recovering from his Achilles injury. As I entered the final mile, coming down Main Street, I came to the intersection with Bowery Street. I looked off to my right and saw the hospital. I thought about how crazy it was that twenty-three years earlier, I had been lying in a bed there, ready to die, knowing that I might never live a full life. I thought of Janet walking into my room with a sausage biscuit. I thought of Dr. Koufos coming into my room and talking with me, trying to get me to eat something, anything, to keep my weight steady. I thought of him pressing a stethoscope to my chest and telling me my heart was strong, and I wondered what he would say on this day, as my heart had powered me through just about twenty miles. As these thoughts swirled in my head, tears poured out of my eyes and my breaths became ragged. I wanted to stop crying because I was coming up to the end of the run, and a lot of people were gathered at the finish line, but I didn't want to stop thinking of my ghosts, not then, not in that space. I had about five hundred feet to go when I dried my eyes off and sucked in a deep breath.

Something happened when I sprinted to catch up with Stu. My legs started cramping. We had already slowed down significantly, and had spent some time walking in the next three miles. But by mile twenty-three, I had to stop. Stu said he had to keep moving because his heel was killing him. He said if he stopped, he would never start again.

"Go," I said. "I'll be right behind you."

I tried to stretch my legs, but the cramps wouldn't let up. One of the Team In Training coaches was there with something to rub on my hamstrings, and that helped a bit. I was able to start running, only this time, I was by myself.

In mile twenty-four, the ghosts joined me. Melissa was there, running like a stork. Dr. Koufos plodded on, talking about my heart and how it had powered me twenty-four and then twenty-five miles and would certainly keep going until the end. Todd was there, hobbling on his one good leg and his one fake leg, cracking jokes about how crazy it was that people would run this far. Tim was there, strong as ever, a swimmer out of water but perfectly able to keep up with me. And Janet was there. She never ran a marathon, or even a race, but she was a runner, and she glided beside me, whispering in my ear that I was almost near the finish line.

My feet shuffled along the road. My legs were so tired I had a hard time picking them up, and this reminded me a bit of how I walked back when I was sick, when even the smallest crack in the sidewalk would send me sprawling to the ground. But I stayed on my feet.

I made a turn and then another turn and all of a sudden, I was in Canal Park and running through the outfield wall. I didn't look up at the hospital, though. I looked forward, toward the finish line. I ran as hard as I could and crossed it almost sprinting.

I walked through the chute and turned right and then I saw it. The hospital. I took a few more steps but then I had to stop and sit down. I needed to look at the hospital and think. I was exhausted and needed to just stop after more than four hours and forty-four minutes of forward movement.

I looked at the hospital and thought about the things I thought about during that training run. I thought of how far I had come, of how magical a journey it had seemed. My ghosts coalesced around me and I felt them all there beside me, congratulating me. I started crying, and a race official and a couple other runners stopped and asked if I was all right.

I'm perfect, I said.

I used to joke after a run that I felt like I was dead, but I've stopped making that joke because it's ridiculous. Every time I finish any run—3 miles, 10 miles, 26.2 miles—no matter how exhausted I might be, I also feel more alive than at any other time.

As I finished that first marathon, as I sat there and stared at the hospital where my life was saved, I thought of the one recurring dream I had during my stay there. I remembered it because of how alive it made me feel, how strong and powerful, at a time when I couldn't even get out of bed to take a bath. It was the baseball dream, the one in which I was running down a hill behind my old elementary school, carrying a baseball glove and ball. I was running fast, so fast. For a long time, I saw this as a dream about baseball because of the glove and ball, and because baseball was my sport. But in the dream, I never actually got to a field to play ball. I just kept running.

I've reframed that dream as one about running now, and I think of it whenever I lace up my shoes and head out for a run, remembering how I wished—when I dreamed it—that I could just keep going, forever. I know I won't keep living, let alone running, forever. But I also know that as long as I am doing either of those things, I will have my ghosts with me. They're not going anywhere, nor do I want them to.

CHAPTER 26

Lessons

My ghosts all have one thing in common. They all spent their lives going above and beyond when it came to caring about others. From the way Dr. Koufos and Janet took care of their patients, both while they were on the clock and off it, to the way Melissa put her heart and soul into maintaining friendships and helping kids with their schoolwork, to the way Todd would work with little kids to show them how the chemotherapy enters their body and how he would make them laugh with his crazy jokes, to how Tim invented a board game when he was just thirteen years old that would help future childhood cancer patients and their parents navigate an uncertain future. They all spent their lives caring for others.

I was not like that, not as a cancer patient and not even as a survivor for a long time. But as I've thought about them for the last twenty years, and recently, as I've gotten to know them through talks with their families, I've realized this is their parting message, their lesson to me.

Care about others. Love everyone in this great, huge, diverse world.

Just before Christmas 2016, the local Fox channel in Cleveland did a story on a fifteen-year-old boy who had leukemia and was being treated at Akron Children's Hospital. He would have to spend Christmas in the hospital, and so his mom was asking viewers to send Christmas cards. She wanted to wallpaper the hospital room in Christmas cheer. I watched the segment a handful of times, and every time the boy was shown, he was in his bed, quiet, seemingly depressed. It was less than a month from the twenty-sixth anniversary of the day I entered Akron Children's, and that boy reminded me of myself in so many ways. I decided to write him a letter and have Lily, my nine-year-old daughter, draw Christmas pictures on the edges.

As I wrote, I told Logan a little bit about myself and what I had gone through. I wanted him to know that he could survive, but I didn't want to tell him he was going to survive. I wanted to tell him some of the things I had learned, things that could help him now.

"I will tell you from experience that you should listen to what your mom tells you," I wrote. "It seems like she is working very hard to help give you a positive attitude in this battle. That is crucial. My mom did the same thing, and when I was sick, it annoyed me to no end, but it helps, ultimately."

I told him I did everything I could to just lie in that bed and hate life, but it was important that he get up, move around. And then I told him what I was only just now starting to realize, after I had spent half of my life writing about being sick.

"This will change you in ways you won't understand for decades," I wrote, "but that's not a bad thing."

"So why did I survive?

I asked Pam that question one day when I was visiting the clinic and looking at my medical records.

"Good question," she said. "I don't know."

"Why do you think I did?"

Pam looked at me.

"I never cared about why I got sick," I continued. "I cared about, why did I live when people like Melissa or Todd didn't."

"It's because the disease they had," Pam said.

She was right about this. I was a very sick patient, that much is true. But I was also a very sick patient with a disease that was more easily treatable than anything Melissa, Todd, Tim, Dr. Koufos, or Janet had. My cancer was in my blood. Their cancers were in the very tissues of their body. Solid tumors are more difficult to treat than some rampant, insane, mutant blood cells. I never considered this until Pam brought it up.

But she went on.

"Why are any of us here?" she said. "It's a real spiritual question, but it's one that survivors wrestle with. It's called survivor's guilt."

Pam told me about another patient she knew, someone who had come along after me. He was one of three patients who all had the same disease, and they were all getting bone marrow transplants around the same time. They were all within a couple years of each other, age-wise.

"The other two kids died," Pam said, "and, not only on the days that it happened, but for a long time afterward, he was just a wreck mentally."

Why do some patients die and others survive?

"If we could answer that question, nobody would die," Pam said.

She's right, of course. Death is perhaps the most natural part of life. It starts and then it stops, and we never know when that will actually happen. It could happen when we are five years old or when we are fifteen or when we are ninety-five. It's just a fact, one that I learned when I was a teenager, when I thought I was immortal, when the only thing that would send me into despair was finding out a girl didn't like me.

I know I'm going to die at some point, just as Melissa knew she was going to die and Todd knew he was going to die and Dr. Koufos knew he was going to die. And just as I know I'm going to die, I also know that I will live on in the minds and hopefully hearts of other people, just as my ghosts have lived on with me. As I get older, with each year farther and farther away from 1991, I try to think less about the unfairness of it all because that's really not the point, right? Instead, I've started thinking about how I could live in a way that would make Dr. Koufos proud, make him feel like his efforts were not wasted on that sick and dying fifteen-year-old so long ago.

"The problem with you guys is you don't know how to be well," Pam said. "You should be well. . . . Maybe you honor those people by living a good life, and not forgetting how fortunate you are and being grateful every day. Honor those people by not forgetting them, by telling their stories."

I don't believe in the type of ghosts you see on TV and in the movies, the spectral kind that float through the air. I don't believe that humans can get trapped between dimensions, between life and the afterlife, because I don't believe in an afterlife. For me, the only way we can live on after we're dead is in the memories of those who knew us. We can live in the hearts and brains of those we leave behind. I believe in the power of stories, and how stories of those who are dead can keep them with us, can spread them out to others, so they will know the ones we cared about. If we all tell enough stories, we can all live forever.

I've been writing about having leukemia since just about the time I stopped chemotherapy treatments. It invades just about everything I write. When I look back on a lot of what I've written over the course of my life, going all the way back to my first essay, a piece I wrote for a contest in *Guideposts*

Magazine (I didn't win), to the initial pieces I wrote in my master of fine arts program's creative writing workshops, to the pieces I've written for national outlets like SB Nation, one thing is usually consistent: I am always referring to those who impacted my life while I was a cancer patient. In that very first piece, Dr. Koufos, Melissa, and Tim were still alive, but Todd, Janet, and Terri and so many others had already died. For a long time, I didn't understand why my illness was all I could write about, but now I understand that I needed other people to know about them. Even then, I was trying to keep their memories alive.

It's only now, nearly twenty-four years after I took my final chemotherapy pill, that I can see that I have a duty as a survivor. I am a survivor who can write and who can remember, and so now, when I ask myself the question, *Why did I survive?* I've decided it's to tell the stories of my ghosts, to make sure others know about those who didn't survive.

Kathy Koufos told me that when her husband died, her heart was shattered into a million pieces. But on the night of the memorial, the one when I read my loving and yet angry essay, the night parent after parent stood up and told story after story about Dr. Koufos, whether he saved their child's life or not, she said something magical happened.

"Every story felt like one of those million pieces was getting put back," she said. "And it was such a valuable experience."

Stories have value. I am grateful that I have stories to tell. The stories I have about Dr. Koufos, Janet, Melissa, Todd, Tim, and all the others are little puzzle pieces that when put together help me understand why I am still here, why I still think about them, and why I will never forget them.

Acknowledgements

This book is a testament to Akron Children's Hospital, for which I will always hold a special place in my heart. So many of the people who worked to save my life in 1991 are still working there, and many of them helped many years later as I tried to understand everything I had gone through. They include Pam Jones, Theresa Borodin, and Nancy Carst. There are also many people who don't appear in this book, but who played a role in making me who I am today, including Char Maxen, Dr. Mohammad Talaizadeh (Dr. Talai to us patients), and a bunch of nurses who I only know their first names, like Joan, Beth, and Jeanne. There is another nurse who didn't show up in this story, but I would be remiss if I didn't mention him. John Perebzak was my second shift nurse one day, and he gave me a 1980 Topps Rickey Henderson rookie baseball card to add to my collection. I keep that card framed and in my office and will never part with it. Also, the public relations team has been amazing and has helped me tell these stories in other forms many times over.

Thanks to the families of my ghosts for being willing to talk with me. I know it isn't easy to talk about someone you miss so much, but your stories about Dr. Koufos, Janet, Melissa, Todd, and Tim will live on forever with me and hopefully everyone who reads this book. Thank you Bill and Joan Seitz, Jack Snyder, Kathy and Kosta Koufos, Denny Forrer, Vanessa Corinealdi, Christine Domer, Louise Lanning, and Jim Lanning. And thanks to Brad Rader for putting me in touch with Kosta.

I have been thinking about this book and talking about this book and writing this book for almost twenty years. As such, there are more people to thank than I could ever possibly name. This all started when I was an undergraduate and taking classes with Joe Mackall and Daniel Lehman at Ashland University, because they were the ones that showed me these experiences could be written about. Then there was grad school at the University of North Carolina Wilmington, where I finally produced a book-length manuscript under the tutelage of David Gessner, Philip Gerard, Wendy Brenner, Sarah Messner, Rebecca Lee, Karen Bender, Clyde Edgerton, and so many more.

Along the way, a great number of people have read bits and pieces of this book, or previous versions of this book, and have given me excellent feedback and encouraged me to keep plugging away, including Andrea Barilla, Stephanie Kist, Valerie Due, and James Sheeler.

I spent six years in the Journalism and Digital Media Department at AU, working with the most amazing colleagues and friends in an environment that will likely never be duplicated. They listened to me talk and rant and more about many things, including this story, so thanks to Gretchen Dworznik, Tim McCarty, Steve Suess, Dave McCoy, and John Skrada. And thanks to the English Department at Fairfield University, which made sure I had the resources necessary to finish this book.

Thanks to Mike Sager and The Sager Group for taking this project on. And thanks to Glenn Stout, who took an essay I wrote on speculation in 2015, helped make it better, and then made sure thousands and thousands of people read it.

Thank you to Mom and Dad, for what you did for me when I was sick and for everything that came after that, especially your willingness to talk about these dark years. Thanks to John and Jim as well.

One person has been by my side, nonstop, since I started writing about having cancer twenty years ago, and that is my amazing, smart, and beautiful wife, Alyssa. Thank you for being there and for having the confidence in me that one day this could be done. You also gave me Emery and Lily, who in so many ways provided additional inspiration to tell this story.

About the Author

Matt Tullis is an assistant professor of digital journalism and English at Fairfield University. He is the host and producer of Gangrey: The Podcast and is an associate editor for *River Teeth: A Journal of Nonfiction Narrative*. He has an MFA from the University of North Carolina Wilmington and has been noted in *The Best American Sports Writing* three times, and *The Best American Essays* once. He lives with his wife and two children in Newtown, Connecticut.

About the Publisher

The Sager Group was founded in 1984. In 2012 it was chartered as a multi-media artists' and writers' consortium, with the intent of empowering those who create art—an umbrella beneath which makers can pursue, and profit from, their craft directly, without gatekeepers.

TSG publishes books; ministers to artists and provides modest grants; and produces documentary, feature, and commercial films. By harnessing the means of production, The Sager Group helps artists help themselves. For more information, please see www.TheSagerGroup.Net.

CPSIA information can be obtained
at www.ICGtesting.com
Printed in the USA
LVOW11s1344041017
551162LV00001B/35/P